D0443321

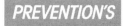

PREVENTION'S

LOSE WEIGHT

GUIDEBOOK

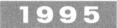

1995

BEST NEW WAYS
TO DROP POUNDS,
TIGHTEN YOUR
TUMMY AND
TONE UP...
PERMANENTLY

EDITED BY MARK BRICKLIN
AND GALE MALESKEY OF *PREVENTION* MAGAZINE

RODALE

Rodale Press, Emmaus, Pennsylvania

Notice

This book is intended as a reference volume only, not as a medical manual. The information given here is designed to help you make informed decisions about your health. It is not intended as a substitute for any treatment that may have been prescribed by your doctor. If you suspect that you have a medical problem, we urge you to seek competent medical help.

ISBN 0–87596–238–6 hardcover
ISSN 1060–9385

Distributed in the book trade by St. Martin's Press

2   4   6   8   10   9   7   5   3   hardcover

OUR MISSION

We publish books that empower people's lives.

RODALE 🌱 BOOKS

Prevention's Lose Weight Guidebook 1995 Editorial and Design Staff

Contributors:

Bob Anderson; Liz Applegate, Ph.D.; Gwenda Blair; Jan Bresnick; Lisa Delaney; Valerie Fahey; Barb Fritz; Mark Golin; Greg Gutfeld; Bruce Henstell; David Higdon; Chris Hill; Anita Hirsch, R.D.; Janet S. Klosko, Ph.D.; Richard Laliberte; Jeff Meade; Linda Miller; Judith Olney; Cathy Perlmutter; Stephen Perrine; Jean Rogers; David Schardt; Porter Shimer; Maggie Spilner; Sharon Stocker; Judith Stone; Jim Thornton; Margo Trott; Jeffrey E. Young, Ph.D.; David Zinczenko

Managing Editor: Sharon Faelten

Executive Editor, *Prevention* Magazine: Emrika Padus

Cover and Book Designers: Lisa Nawaz, Lynn N. Gano

Studio Manager: Joe Golden

Layout Designer: Carl Nielsen/Bookhead Studio

Technical Artist: Kristen Page Morgan

Permissions: Anita Small

Copy Editor: Stacey Ann Cortese

Office Personnel: Roberta Mulliner, Julie Kehs, Bernadette Sauerwine, Mary Lou Stephen

Prevention Magazine Health Books

Editor-in-Chief, Rodale Books: Bill Gottlieb

Executive Editor: Debora A. Tkac

Art Director: Jane Colby Knutila

Research Manager: Ann Gossy Yermish

Copy Manager: Lisa D. Andruscavage

Contents

Fast-Start Tips to Shed Pounds and Keep Them Off

De-stress Your Tummy Away

Cope with Cravings

Use Muscle-Building to Banish Fat

Striding to Slimness

Stay Psyched

Slash the Fat, Save the Flavor

Introduction

Staying lean pays off big when it comes to a long, healthy life.

When we're 18 or 25 or even 35, we have lots of motivation to stay slim and trim. We want to squeeze into our skin-tight jeans, get ogled at the beach, admire what we see when we look in the mirror. In other words, we want to look good to attract mates. That's our biological imperative, and whether we like it or not, in our society, for most people, sexual attraction is equated with physical attraction. And physical attraction is equated with slimness. Some of us go to extremes to achieve shapes society considers attractive.

So what happens when we get older, get married, get comfortable and, hopefully, become more accepting of ourselves the way we are? For most people, the motivation to lose weight drops off, and the pounds creep on. When we do diet, the weight we lose always seems to find its way back.

That wouldn't be so bad if we could be fat and happy—and healthy. But eventually, those pounds catch up with many of us. We all know that being overweight contributes to the development of heart disease, but researchers have discovered that people who are overweight also have a higher-than-normal risk of a long list of ailments. Some—like diabetes, high blood pressure, breast cancer, colon cancer, prostate cancer, arthritis and back pain—you've probably heard about. Other weight-related problems—sleep disorders, fertility problems, gallstones and carpal tunnel syndrome—will come as a surprise to you. Any one of those ailments can put a serious damper on our quality of life and, in some cases, our quantity of life.

While escaping weight-related maladies may be a powerful motivator, it's still a negative one. So consider this. Time and again, *Prevention* magazine readers who've lost weight tell us all the good that's come of their accomplishments. They've been able to stop taking blood pressure or diabetes medication, and they're glad to be rid of the unpleasant side effects. Losing weight, they tell us, has enabled them to avoid surgery, reduce arthritis pain and sleep better. Some say they have more stamina than they've had in years and that their zest for life is stronger than ever. One middle-aged man even reported that he'd developed the sex drive of a 16-year-old lifeguard—to his wife's amazement.

The common denominator: They all feel better—and feel better about themselves—once they get their weight to where it should be.

How did they do it? By following the kind of advice you'll find in this book. Advice on how to exercise at home without fancy equipment and use nature to help you relax. Tips on how to resist cravings, exercise to boost your metabolism and create low-fat recipes that sacrifice absolutely nothing in taste. Suggestions for making smart on-the-go eating choices and walking away stress and pounds at the same time.

It's *Prevention*'s unique combination of information and inspiration that leads to weight-loss success, without a sense of sacrifice or deprivation. It's knowledge you can use to improve your life.

—*The Editors*

Part One

Fast-Start Tips to Shed Pounds and Keep Them Off

Year of the Svelte:
Lose a Pound a Week

Use these fat-fighting tips to drop pounds, year-round.

When it comes to weight loss, success is in the details. Whether it's finding a tastier way to dress up a nonfat food, making an exercise a little bit more effective or marshaling more motivation to get you going, it's the little things that matter. And those little things are just what you need to drop the steady one pound a week that experts agree is the safest, healthiest and most effective schedule for permanent weight loss.

That's why we've given you 52 realistic ways to drop that one pound. Some tips take just seconds to do; others require that you make minor adjustments to things you're already doing. There are tips for the dinner table, tips for the exercise room and tips that can make it just a little easier to keep your motivation at an all-time high. Use a few; use them all.

Fat-Skimming Secrets

If you already skip the pats of butter on your muffin and bag the cream in your morning coffee, you know small changes can slowly nickel-and-dime the weight away. Here are a few more edible moves to keep you up to fat-fighting snuff.

Put the beans to the buns. Already using extra-lean ground beef or turkey in your burgers? Try substituting mashed pinto beans or black beans for half the meat. You'll boost fiber and flavor while slashing fat in half.

Dash, then dine. Do you eat and run? Just reverse the order. Eating after exercising may help ignite a potent calorie burn. The thermic effect of food, which causes resting metabolic rate to rev up after munching, may get an extra boost in combination with the higher metabolic rate that also occurs after a workout.

Have a pre-exercise snack. Before exercising, it may help to eat, too. Not a meal, mind you, but a snack. Roughly two hours before working out, have a plain bagel or a piece of fruit. It can give you some extra energy and alertness while holding off the hunger gremlins until you get home. If you go too many hours without eating, you are more likely to gorge at that post-exercise meal.

Try some "green" protein. If you've given up meat, you don't have to give up protein. Try the top two fresh vegetable sources: lima beans and green peas. A ¾-cup serving of limas has seven grams of protein, while the same amount of peas contains more protein than a whole egg or a tablespoon of peanut butter. You get the body-building protein without the fat.

Review your battle plan. Make a list of five strategies that are most helpful in maintaining your diet success (e.g., eating only low-fat snacks, not buying high-fat snack foods, packing your lunch and so forth). Every month, check the list to be sure that you're doing all those things. "We often experience a subtle falling away from our goals," says Linda Crawford, a certified eating disorders counselor and eating-behavior specialist at Green Mountain at Fox Run in Ludlow, Vermont. "You're able to correct the problem easily within a short period of time if you check what you're doing each month."

Top this spud. You can't get much better than a baked spud, sans the butter pat, topped with nonfat sour cream. But if you're craving a new flavor, try adding a little grated horseradish or applesauce for a lively new topping. Chili sauce is another great nonfat potato pleaser.

"Urge-surf." Generally, after food urges start, they come to a peak and then nosedive. If you can ride that urge, you can save on guilt and pounds. To urge-surf, find an alternative activity—a shower, a walk, a bike ride, anything that's incompatible with eating. "If you spend just five to ten minutes doing this, the urge may go away," says Jonathan Robison, Ph.D., executive co-director, Michigan Center for Preventive Medicine in Lansing. "But don't mistake real hunger for an urge. You still have to eat!"

Don't cook on empty. You know that grocery shopping while hungry is a no-no. The same advice applies to cooking. If you're hungry and surrounded by cooking food, you're bound to nibble through the preparation as well as make more food than you really need. Take the edge off by having a light but satisfying snack before you begin to cook. Slice an apple or melon, or put together a plate of baby carrots, cherry tomatoes and broccoli florets with a bowl of nonfat salad dressing as dip.

Snack as a pack. To keep snacking low-fat but fun, designate a canister or drawer for each member of the family and fill it with their favorite healthy snacks. Then mix them up and share them when it comes time for movie-rental night.

Stick to the rim. In too much of a hurry to read the labels at the supermarket? To ensure you make low-fat choices, stick to the outside aisles. Along the perimeter, you'll find mostly fresh and healthy stuff—breads, fruits, veggies and low-fat dairy products. Venturing into the heart of darkness—the center aisles—may land you in High Fatville.

Go with cocoa. "When you're looking for dessert recipes, choose one that uses cocoa instead of baking chocolate. This can save you about 13 grams of fat for each ounce of baking chocolate. If you can't find a recipe that uses cocoa, combine three tablespoons of cocoa powder with one tablespoon of canola oil, which still saves you 1 to 2 grams of fat for each one-ounce square of baking chocolate in the recipe," says Dayle Hayes, a registered dietitian at Deaconess Medical Center in Billings, Montana. "You can use cocoa to make a low-fat frosting or combine it with fat-free treats like meringues, fresh fruit and frozen yogurt."

Take the "in" out. Researchers have actually studied folks who have to eat out frequently and found that, on the whole, they take in more fat and calories than those who eat at home. Combat this by packing travel snacks to take with you for long trips and flights. If you must hit the burger joints, spy the healthier stuff—grilled chicken (minus the mayo) and salads without the fat-laden dressings. Top the meal off with low- or nonfat frozen yogurt.

Pass on the pat. Still can't let go of butter? Try this strategy: Instead of loading up on butter, try squeezing a fresh lemon over your food.

Do the A.M. shuffle. Put five different low-fat breakfasts on cards. Each morning pick one. That way you can wake up looking forward to a little variety rather than the same old bran. Even better, it can help you sidestep the urge to make a drive-thru detour for egg-and-ham biscuits on the way to work.

Block the midnight binge. Keep fast, healthy foods on hand for those late work nights or sudden cravings. That prevents the desperate grab for anything edible when you are overworked or stressed or just plain have the munchies. Keep pasta and sauce, frozen premade low-fat meals like burritos or chicken and low-fat frozen dinners handy. Cereal and oatmeal, even without milk, are great midnight meals, too.

Keep a diet diary. If you seem to be gaining weight even though you think you're sticking to low-fat foods, try jotting down what you eat for two or three days out of one week. Be sure to include one weekend day. "Sometimes people can really fool themselves about what they're actually taking in," says Denise Marecki, R.D., a nutritionist at the clinical research center at the University of Michigan Hospitals in Ann Arbor. "We kept a log on one person and noticed he tended to eat a lot of fast food while driving. His car actually became a trigger to eat." A short-term log may help identify and target diet-crushing patterns like that.

Eat before you mall. Go to any of the nearby shopping malls, and you'll have to run the gauntlet of tantalizing temptresses—known collectively as the food court. Fill up before you shop, and you'll be less likely to be found munching sweet rolls, slurping shakes and contemplating a plate of nachos.

Slow down. If you're a fast eater who tends to blow through a meal while others are at nibble speed, follow this simple rule: Never have a spoon or fork in your hand as long as there's food in your mouth. You may even start tasting the food more. You also keep pace with the other diners.

Get a gadget. To keep you interested in low-fat cooking, purchase a utensil or gadget, suggests Liz Applegate, Ph.D., a nutritionist at the University of California, Davis, Department of Nutrition. "Try a good set of no-stick cookware. Or get yourself a yogurt maker—it's a great way to add a healthy food to your diet. It can also help you eat more fruits—as toppings."

Try a speedy veggie slicer. "To be honest, when I initially plan to put three or four different vegetables in a salad,

I opt for one because I don't want to chop them," says Dr. Applegate. "But if you whiz them through a machine, you don't have to do anything except eat more veggies."

Share the stove. If you don't have time to prepare healthy foods every night, trade off cooking duties with a friend, says Crawford. Ask a friend who enjoys cooking low-fat to make extras of meals that can be frozen. In exchange for her service, you could do the same.

Get an education. "Check out the food section of your local newspaper and see what kinds of cooking classes are offered, then get a friend to go along," says Dr. Applegate. "Finding a low-fat class would be great—helping you to branch out into new flavors, ideas and combinations."

Pay heed to the hue. Eat in the blue room, not in the red. According to research from the Health, Weight and Stress Clinic at Johns Hopkins Medical Institutions in Baltimore, warm hues like red, yellow and orange make food look better and make people hungrier. Cool colors like blue and gray, though, have the opposite effect.

Fitness Fine-Tuners

If your daily walk is giving you the blahs, try some of these calorie-incinerating, muscle-building and psychological kick-in-the-pants suggestions. They can freshen your workout and drop-kick the pounds. Here are new ways to do old things as well as tips to ignite your fat-burning metabolism by maximizing your muscle.

Protect your sacred time. The first thing you should do every day is schedule your workout. Set time aside and guard it religiously. "No one else is going to do it for you," says Fredrick C. Hagerman, Ph.D., professor of biological sciences at Ohio University in Athens and physiological consultant to the U.S. Olympic rowing team. Let your friends and co-workers know when that special time is.

Review your moves. Periodically, take a look at the written instructions for the exercises you do, if you've gotten such information from a physical therapist or a trainer. Over time, you can stray from the actual technique and forget the right way to do things.

Go a step further and take turns with a friend filming your workouts. Then watch your form and compare it with how the exercise should be done. You may notice mistakes in your form or speed that can reduce the effectiveness of your workout. You can also use video to analyze your walking stride.

Clock in with consistency. If you don't work out at roughly the same time each day, you may be more likely to blow it off. "Your body responds very nicely to habit," says Dr. Hagerman. "Do your best to keep your exercise scheduled at consistent times."

Remember to be eccentric. Because building muscle is one important key to burning fat (muscle is hungry tissue and burns more energy), you need to do it right.

When you're lifting weights, you're also letting weights down. That part of the exercise may seem easy—but it's the key to really building muscle. When you let the weight down (called the eccentric contraction), do it slowly to get the most out of it. Resist the temptation to let the weight down fast. Instead, fight gravity and drop it down slowly with each repetition. That stresses the muscles more, which makes them stronger.

Take lessons. If you're in a rut with running, take swimming lessons. If you're tired of tennis, take lessons for racquetball. It can keep things fresh. "Just trying something different—a dance class, for example—keeps your attitude about exercise positive," says Dr. Applegate.

Drop Danielle Steele books and start pedaling. It's fine to read a book or the morning paper while you pedal on your stationary bike. But you might want to introduce a few extra-tough intervals that allow you to concentrate on your performance rather than the plot. Put the book down and pedal harder. Get your heart and muscles working for one minute. After that interval, resume your regular pace and page turning. You can burn more calories, strengthen the muscles and spice up the activity.

Make a note of your achievements. Better yet, put that note on your bathroom mirror. "Reminding yourself of what you've done is great motivation to keep at it," says Dr. Robison. "It's a simple way to establish a pattern."

Find a friendly adversary. Work out with friends and try to match them for total time of exercise. But don't aim for who is stronger or faster; go by level of commitment instead. "Ask any professional athlete—friendly rivalries make great motivators," says Charles Kuntzleman, Ed.D., national program director for Fitness Finders. It's peaceful one-upmanship.

Observe first. If you want to take an aerobics class to get rid of that belly bulge but you're intimidated by the group activity, go watch a class first and even meet with the instructor. "This may make you more comfortable starting up an unfamiliar activity rather than jumping right in," says Dr. Robison. It may also save you the trouble of entering a class that is too advanced or not demanding enough of your ability.

Step up. A stair-climber machine is a great fat burner—ridding your body of as many as 680 calories per hour—when it's used right. "The range of motion is much larger than what your legs normally do, so try to limit your steps to eight to ten inches in the up and down motion," says Budd Coates, corporate fitness director at Rodale Press and editorial consultant to *Runner's World* magazine. But avoid skimming the surface with tiny steps. "Go almost to the top and almost to the bottom—that'll work the leg muscles to a greater extent," says Coates. "Always keep an erect posture, or you'll begin to crouch and develop a lower back problem."

Watch your toes. On a stair-climber, make sure your knees don't go over your toes. You'll be taking smaller steps, but you'll protect the ligaments in your knees, allowing you to exercise longer and burn more calories.

Keep your hands off. You can hold the rails of the stair-climber, but only for balance. Don't use them as support or slump over the machine like it's closing time at the local saloon—you'll diminish the total calorie burn.

Nix the numbness. To prevent your midfoot or toes from becoming numb on a stair-climber, which can abruptly end a workout, loosen your shoe or move your toes as you go along. Tense and relax them while you step. "You can also stop and take a break so the circulation returns," says Coates.

Make it social. Plan social gatherings around activities that don't involve food and instead target those that involve movement. Roller skating, ice skating, tennis, hiking and group workouts at the gym are all great ways to catch up with friends while burning off a little fat.

Know thy row. Rowing's total-body workout offers a potent calorie burn—about 440 calories per hour. "People often think of it as a resistance form of exercise, though, and burn themselves out," says Dr. Hagerman. "If you want an aerobic workout, stick to a rowing ergometer with its free-moving wheel as well as a sliding seat that uses the large leg muscles instead of relying solely on the upper body."

A beginner's workout should amount to no more than four 3-minute bouts with a minute of rest in between each. Over time, work up to two continuous bouts of 15-minute periods. Then work up to one 30-minute block and alternate it with your other favorite aerobic exercise.

Try a no-fuss muscle workout. When you're standing in a checkout line, you can tighten the gluteal muscles of your fanny or tighten your abdominal muscles. "Those little motions aren't going to replace really good training, but they help strengthen musculature in a surprisingly easy manner," says Dr. Kuntzleman.

Ski easy. An indoor cross-country skiing machine is great for trimming down—but don't make it tough on yourself. "Adjust the tension of the arm handles and skis so they are similar, and don't make it so tough that you tire quickly," says Coates. "The exercise needs to be continuous aerobic activity in order to burn calories. Having the machine at a high resistance keeps you from doing it for a considerable amount of time."

Get down. If you like burning your calories on a stationary bike but it's bothersome to your back, try the recumbent version. It doesn't burn quite the same amount of calories, but it allows you to sit back in a low-slung, reclining position that helps protect your back.

Sweat with cinema. Camp a VCR near your stationary bicycle, treadmill or the indoor aerobic device of your choice and watch your favorite movies. "Exercise seems to flow much better when you are watching something you're interested in rather than watching a talking head from the news or a talk show," says Dr. Kuntzleman. "Target your interests, and you'll find you may last longer and enjoy it as well."

Sleep in your duds. Go to bed with your workout clothes on. "That gives you a head start in the morning," says Dr. Kuntzleman. By wearing a shirt and even sweat pants to sleep, getting out of a warm bed in the morning isn't such a shocker. Don't try this with Lycra biking shorts, however.

Give your muscles a break. More muscle means a higher metabolism. That means you burn more calories. But in order to have more muscle, you need rest. Your body must recuperate in order to get strong and stay healthy. "The optimum rest period for one muscle group is roughly 48 hours," says Dr. Hagerman. "Never target the same muscle group two days in a row."

Grab a buzz. Something as simple as a haircut may incite you to work out more. A wash-and-wear clip may allow you to work out at lunch without a lot of fuss after.

Throw your shoes in the trunk—now! It takes only a minute, and if you do it now, you'll be prepared to walk during your lunch hour. You may want to take a minute to call a co-worker and ask him to do the same.

Give yourself a spread. Having one fixed goal to work toward can discourage you if you miss it. Instead, give yourself a space to succeed. Don't tell yourself you're going to work out five times a week—instead pencil in "three to five times." "Perfectionism can really kill an exercise program or a healthy diet," says Dr. Kuntzleman.

Sweat to sound. Use music in rhythm with your workout. "No matter what the exercise is, if the beat is in pace with your body, it can be very helpful," says Dr. Kuntzleman. "It allows you to disassociate yourself from the repetitiveness you might get from regular exercise." Indoors, a personal radio with headphones can be a boredom stopper.

Keep treading steady. If you like walking on a treadmill to burn fat in wintertime but always feel off balance or even dizzy, there may be one simple remedy. "Don't look side to side, even if you're talking to someone," says Coates. "You'll tend to sway and then lose your balance." Always look forward. If you watch TV, keep the tube in front of you.

Split it up. "Thirty minutes of sustained exercise each day is great, but it may not be possible on a particularly hectic day," says Dr. Robison. If you think you have to skip a workout because you just can't find that 30-minute block of time in one chunk, look for smaller bites. You can still get the benefits if you simply split that block into three

10-minute shots—and do the three in one day. Try a brisk walk in the morning, at lunch and after dinner.

Make a bet. Try exercising—Vegas-style. In a study at Michigan State University in East Lansing, people who bet $40 that they could stick with their programs for six months had a 97 percent success rate. Less than 20 percent of those who didn't bet stuck to their routines.

Be aware. To keep an endurance workout from becoming stale, be aware of what's going on inside you. While exercising aerobically, your heart and lungs are processing more oxygen. "Visualize your coronary blood vessels dilating and working, with the red blood cells picking up more oxygen, transporting it to other cells," says Dr. Kuntzleman. "I notice I run better this way. With disease, many patients are told to visualize immune cells fighting the illness. You may not be ill, but you can use the same strategy here."

—Greg Gutfeld with Michele Toth

Find the Body Weight That's Best for You

Use a blend of ingenuity and exercise to refine your daily calorie balance.

In theory, the energy equation that reflects your body weight should be very simple. The number of calories you take in minus the number of calories you burn should equal the three digits staring up at you from the scale every morning. But it's usually not that easy. And as a result, many people struggle to achieve a precarious balance.

Small wonder. Calorie-burning potential is partially predetermined—a product of genetics and gender—so it exists outside of the energy equation. But that's only half the scoop. The other half, which is far more heartening, holds that you can help your body to burn calories faster. The trick is to fiddle with what and when you eat and when and how you exercise. Only then can you circumvent your pesky genetics and lose the weight you want to.

Facts and Figures

The calories you ingest by eating and drinking are referred to as calories in. Those you burn by doing anything from brushing your teeth to running a marathon are called calories out. To maintain your body weight, calories in must equal calories out. To lose weight, you must reduce calories in and maintain calories out, maintain calories in and increase calories out or reduce calories in and increase calories out. As you can see, this is where things get a little sticky.

Three factors contribute to calorie burning. The most important is your resting metabolic rate, which is the amount of energy your body uses for basic functions such as breathing, thinking and pumping blood and oxygen through your body. For most people, this accounts for 60 to 75 percent of all of the calories they burn each day, or about 1,100 to 2,000 calories.

The speed of your resting metabolic rate depends primarily on your body composition. The more muscle—or "lean body mass"—you have, the faster your metabolic rate. Women by nature have proportionately more body fat and less muscle than men, which is why they have metabolic rates roughly 10 percent lower than men. Metabolic rates for both men and women drop as they grow older, due in part to the loss of muscle mass that accompanies the aging process.

As the second factor in the calories-out part of the energy equation, activity accounts for 15 to 35 percent of the calories you burn every day. Any activity you engage in—walking, bicycling or just plain fidgeting—burns calories above your resting metabolic rate. Of course, brisk walking eats up more calories than fidgeting, so this factor will vary depending on the types of activities you do and how long you do them.

The third and least significant of the calorie-burning components is the energy your body expends processing food. Digesting, transporting and storing the fat, protein and carbohydrates is hard work, accounting for 75 to 200 of the calories your body burns each day. While this thermic effect of food, as it is called, usually represents no more than 10 percent of the total number of calories you use daily, small fluctuations can add up over time. Some people who are very overweight, for instance, have low thermic effect values, which may contribute to their tendency to gain weight.

Surefire Solutions

As you can see, your body burns calories naturally—up to a point. Following are a few ways you can increase the burn and balance a complex caloric equation that may have your body stumped.

Stay active. Exercising regularly (by walking or doing strength-training or aerobics, for instance) helps you to boost your metabolism and regulate your food intake. When you don't exercise, your body loses touch with its own internal regulatory system. Hunger signals and feelings of fullness aren't as pronounced. And as a result, your eating patterns and body weight tend to fluctuate more.

Maximize the afterburn. Exercising doesn't just boost calorie burning during your workouts; it increases it afterward, too. For up to 24 hours after a workout, your resting metabolic rate is faster than normal, burning anywhere from 50 to a few hundred calories more than usual. While this may not sound like much, it adds up. In fact, exercise afterburn could save you the equivalent of two to five pounds of fat over several months. And that's nothing to sneeze at.

Because afterburn is simply the body working hard (and expending calories) to rebuild spent fuel stores, repair damaged muscle fibers and normalize your body temperature, the longer or harder you exercise, the greater the afterburn. Take full advantage of this phenomenon by increasing the amount of time you exercise as well as the intensity of your workouts every once in a while. For instance, once or twice a week, try carrying light weights in each hand as you zip through your normal walking workout.

Run, then eat. Eating soon after you exercise may boost calorie burning. Various studies have shown that thermic effect is greater after exercise. Since your body burns extra calories after you work out and your resting metabolic rate revs up immediately after you eat, following a workout with a meal may boost calorie burning that much more.

Unfortunately, thermic effect may not rise after exercise in individuals at either end of the activity-level spectrum. Although the reason is unclear, very unfit individuals and highly trained athletes don't seem to burn extra calories after eating.

Pump up. Strength-training will help you to increase your lean body mass and rev up your resting metabolic rate. How? By building muscle. Since muscle tissue requires more calories to sustain itself than fat tissue does, your body will expend extra calories if it becomes more muscular.

Eat up. Calorie skimpers know all too well the frustration of a slowed metabolism. And if you're a regular exerciser, you can afford to eat more than others. After all, your body will burn more calories if you boost your food intake. And if you take in more calories to offset the calories you burn while walking or swimming, your body will expend that much more energy on "shipping and handling" all of the incoming calories.

Eat often. In a study of lean women, 75 percent reported eating at least four times a day. And we know that people who struggle with unwanted pounds are often meal skippers. Whether this practice leads to a weight problem by prompting overeating at other meals or whether missing meals is an eating habit that develops in an effort to lose weight is still unclear. The bottom line, however, is not—eat small meals often.

Skim the fat. A diet composed of lots of carbohydrates (more than 60 percent) and little fat (less than 25 percent) increases calorie burning. Why? Because your body processes and stores fat more efficiently than it does carbohydrates. In fact, when given a choice, the body prefers to store fat rather than to burn it immediately for energy.

Carbohydrates, on the other hand, are either burned quickly or stored as fuel for muscle or as fat. And because the body doesn't store carbohydrates very efficiently, your thermic effect rises when you eat them, burning more calories.

Thermic effect is lower after a high-fat meal than after a high-carbohydrate meal because it costs the body very little to move fat from the intestines into fat storage. Not so with carbohydrates. As a result, you burn fewer calories while you sleep after eating a high-fat meal than after eating a meal packed with carbohydrates. Again, a few calories here and there add up over time and can lead to unwanted pounds or much-desired weight loss. The choice is up to you.

—*Liz Applegate, Ph.D.*

Ten Surefire Tricks to Help You Stay on Your Diet

Diet expert Dr. Stephen Gullo reveals the secrets of his clients' success.

Most diets are a lot like death and taxes—you have to deal with them, but rarely do you feel that you've come out on the winning side. No matter how innovative the diet, the bottom line seems the same: So long as you wear handcuffs to the table, you'll take off weight. But the pounds come right back as soon as you remove the shackles.

The problem, says Stephen Gullo, Ph.D., psychologist and diet guru to many of Manhattan's rich and famous, is that with most diets you lose only the pounds—not the reasons behind them. The way Dr. Gullo sees it, a diet is akin to an iceberg. Spotting the tip of an iceberg is easy; so is seeing the extra weight you want to shed. What causes trouble is the part you can't see. With an iceberg, it is what is hidden below the waterline; with a diet, it is all the reasons that led you to put too much food in your mouth in the first place.

Rigid rules won't keep off those extra pounds. Knowing how much fat is in a french fry won't do it either. Weight control is not about willpower or character or even calories. It's about genes—that is, what your body is programmed to burn and what it is programmed to store as fat. It is also about cultural background—what you were raised to think of as tasty and comforting. And it is about the food habits that you've built up over a lifetime. As a result, the only diet that has a chance of working is one tailored to individual eating patterns—the what, where, when and why of you and food. Only after you've established what Dr. Gullo calls your eating print (EP) will you be able to start losing weight for good.

Here are his guidelines on how to figure out your own EP.

What. Most people with weight problems are eating too much of something. The trick is to figure out exactly what. It can be anything from candy and cookies to cheeses, rich sauces, even bread sticks. Whatever it is, it's your "trigger food," and ordinary calorie counting won't help you control your consumption of it, because you don't eat it in units of one. The critical number here is not the 60 calories in, say, 1 chocolate chip cookie but the multiples of 60 that make up the calories in the 10 to 15 cookies you'll scarf up in a single sitting.

Often the problem is not the specific food but the type. Finger foods like cookies, bonbons, pretzels, popcorn and even grapes or cherries are especially risky. They are not served in individual portions and thus lack what Dr. Gullo calls a finish line, so your fingers keep reaching until the bowl, box or plate is empty.

If you can't figure out what your trigger food is, don't give up. You may not have one. Sometimes, because of personal body chemistry or age, people simply don't metabolize certain foods efficiently. If, for example, you are eating only pasta with low-fat sauce and you're still gaining weight, you probably don't burn up starch very well.

Where. For most women, their own kitchens are the most dangerous place. Men are "equal-opportunity eaters" who eat—and overeat—anything, anywhere, anytime. By contrast, women eat small servings in public and overdo it at home, often on food they ostensibly bought for their families.

A surprising number of people eat standing up, and it can be as dangerous as eating finger foods. When you're snacking off the shelf or out of the refrigerator, there's no finish line. Worse, you're likely to assume that bites taken while you're on your feet somehow don't count as much as those taken when you're sitting down.

When. The most vulnerable time for many is what Dr. Gullo calls the first ten minutes. This can occur when you get home from work, when you've just arrived at a party or a restaurant or right after guests leave and you're cleaning up. Your guard is down, it's only a bite, an hors d'oeuvre, a snack, a bread basket—you're too hungry to wait, and these excuses and more come to mind. The important point is that no matter when you eat it, food is still food, and for most people, it's the food eaten before or after official meals that puts on the weight.

Why. At least some of the time, people eat because they're hungry. But many overeat because they believe it is possible to "have it all"—to eat everything and stay thin. Ask yourself whether you are assuming you can have whatever you want without paying the price.

People also overeat because they are unhappy. Of course, not all weight problems are emotional problems—you don't have to be crazy to be crazy about a cookie. But if you have a history of weight problems, it's important to determine whether you're consistently overeating as a way of dealing with stress or depression or anger.

Weight control will never be easy—but it will always be easier than being fat. According to a study of 96 women at the University of Arizona in Tuscon and research findings from the past three decades, lower body weight is linked to a significantly reduced incidence of serious disease and to longer lives. Whether or not thinner is aesthetically or politically desirable, there can be no argument that it is healthier. That, says Dr. Gullo, is reason enough to pursue it.

Knowing your EP is only the first step. Next comes learning how to adapt your own diet accordingly. Unlike most diet doctors, Dr. Gullo steers away from particular menus or magic bullets. In his view, the only successful diet is one that's never over. Real success requires a permanent change in eating habits and thinking. Accordingly, instead of listing amounts and ingredients, he focuses on the notion of weight control as a management skill with specific techniques.

Here are his basic tips for keeping weight off for good.

Say good-bye to trigger foods. Once you've identified your trigger food, eliminate it. If you haven't already learned how to have just a little, you're not going to learn now. Don't con yourself into believing that you can control it. You can't. If your problem is food supposedly bought for others but—somehow—consumed by you, don't put it in your shopping cart. If it's something other than a trigger food, something your body doesn't metabolize well, stop eating it. Thus, if eating bread and pasta puts on the pounds, switch to animal-based protein and little or no starch.

Don't even think about it. Thinking about a trigger food is the first step toward eating it. Looking at it or smelling it are further steps along the way. Having it available creates craving; having a half-dozen varieties on your shelf creates even more craving. Remember the frequency/quantity principle, also known as the FQ principle, which simply states that once you increase the frequency of a trigger food, the quantity will increase as well. Say you have a weakness for pretzels and so you have just one. Your very success at holding yourself to one will encourage you to have another one the next day, two the day after and so on.

Don't expect food to solve emotional problems.
Somewhere deep inside, says Dr. Gullo, when people are
troubled, they still look to food for comfort and to feel better. In reality, food can provide only temporary relief, and
overeating will simply make you overweight as well as
unhappy. Whether you gorge yourself with cookies or
not, you'll still have to deal with the curveballs life throws
at you.

Never eat when you're hungry. Contrary to most diet
advice, Dr. Gullo says flatly that you should never go to
dinner on an empty stomach. If you drink a glass of tomato
juice or eat a piece of fruit or some diet Jell-O beforehand,
you'll be in charge, not your taste buds.

Use premenstrual precaution. Many women crave
chocolate just before their periods because of hormonal
changes. Rather than bingeing and gaining, try nonfat substitutes, such as Alba chocolate shakes or Weight Watchers
chocolate mousse pops. Likewise, women who have a yen
for salty items before their periods should try low-calorie
versions—pickles rather than pretzels or crackers, for example. If you have major hunger pangs during these few days,
schedule a fourth meal; it will help you avoid indiscriminate
snacking.

If you're a slow loser, eat green and white. If you feel
like you're not getting anywhere, don't give up. Instead,
switch to a green (vegetables and salads) and white
(chicken or turkey) menu. It can provide a jump start and
thus a boost to your morale. This is not the best diet to live
on, but it is one of the best for losing weight.

Aim for your personal best weight. Rather than feeling like a failure because you can't get down to an ideal
number on a chart, focus on the lowest weight you can
maintain given your history and lifestyle. As in sports, don't
worry about the Olympic record; just go for what Dr. Gullo
calls your personal thin.

Remember that cravings are not commands. Strong as they sometimes are, food cravings do pass—often in only a few minutes. The best way to wait a craving out is not to fight it head-on but to distract yourself with something you enjoy, such as a phone call to a friend.

Don't use slips as excuses to eat more. Everyone is going to overeat once in a while, but that doesn't have to mean a permanent defeat. Gobbling a handful of cookies is a disaster only if you let that be an excuse to have two handfuls the next day. Consider your mistakes to be learning experiences.

Don't rely on exercise to bail you out. No matter how many leg lifts you do, your legs will never go as fast as your fingers. Exercise will burn up some calories, but it's not a trade-off for indulging in too many trigger foods. What exercise does give you is a positive awareness of your body and a sense of having control over your life. It is also an outlet for the emotional distress that can lead to overeating.

There's no such thing as a never-say-no diet. Having it all doesn't exist in life, and it doesn't exist on the table. "Not being able to eat anything, anywhere, anytime is not a terrible fate, but reality," says Dr. Gullo. "The sooner people accept this, the easier effective weight control will be."

—Gwenda Blair

The Truth about Dieting

Discerning fact from fiction can help you pare down.

You'd think people would know a lot more about weight, considering how much energy most of us spend worrying about it. Yet how many of you can pick out the one statement among the following three that's false?

1. It's easier for men to lose weight than women.
2. Gaining weight in your belly is more dangerous than gaining weight in your thighs.
3. It's better to gain weight as you get older.

Not easy, huh? The only false one is number three. Actually, there are a ton of false ones. So read on, as we explode some common misconceptions about weight and weight loss.

Myth: *Americans are getting leaner.*

Truth: We're getting fatter. Despite health clubs on every corner, swarms of people out jogging, weight-loss centers in shopping malls and hospitals and all the new low-calorie and low-fat foods, the percentage of Americans who are overweight is increasing. That's especially true for people who

25

Getting Waist-to-Hip Ratio

Are you an apple or a pear?

Most men are apples. They're wider around the belly and chest. Most women are pears. They're wider around the hips and thighs.

Apples have a far greater risk of developing heart disease, high blood pressure, high blood sugar and high insulin. Sadly, the only thing about them that's lower is their level of high-density lipoproteins (HDLs), or good cholesterol. And what do pears suffer more from? Varicose veins and problems in the knees, which have to support their heavier hips.

You can't go from being an apple to being a pear or vice versa. But since most people lose weight from their upper bodies faster than from their lower bodies, you can become less of an apple or a thinner pear simply by taking off a few pounds. Your goal should be to have a waist-to-hip ratio below 0.95 (men) or 0.85 (women). Here's how to measure yours. All you'll need is a tape measure.

Using the chart opposite, make a mark along the left-hand scale next to your waist measurement (it's the smallest measurement below your rib cage and above your belly button). Then make another mark along the right-hand scale next to

are already overweight and for younger women.

People who aren't overweight are most likely to become so between the ages of 34 and 45.

Myth: *The most unhealthy thing about being overweight is the stress it puts on your heart.*

Truth: That's only one of your troubles. Excess weight raises insulin levels, which can lead to diabetes and high

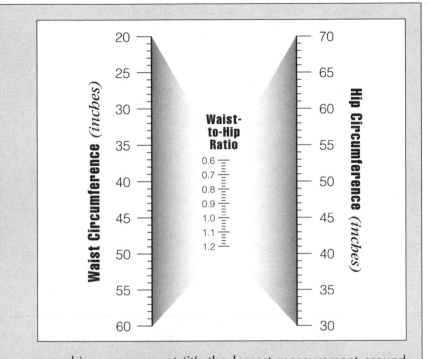

your hip measurement (it's the largest measurement around the widest part of your buttocks). Draw a line connecting the marks. The point at which the line crosses the waist-to-hip ratio scale down the middle of the chart is your ratio.

blood pressure. It also raises the level of low-density lipo-proteins (LDLs), the bad cholesterol, and lowers the level of high-density lipoproteins (HDLs), the good cholesterol, and that means an increased risk of heart disease.

What's more, if you're obese (see "Oh, My, BMI" on page 30), your body's hormonal balance could be thrown out of whack. If you're a woman, that increases your risk of breast and endometrial cancer and menstrual irregularities. And everyone runs a greater risk of developing gallstones, arthritis and even sleep disorders.

Perhaps the most unhealthy thing about being overweight is that you don't feel like exercising. And that's a real killer.

Myth: *A pound is a pound, whether it's on my hips or my belly.*

Truth: Extra weight in the chest and belly is far more unhealthy than extra weight around the hips and thighs. Hip and thigh fat is stable. Once it's there, it tends to stay put. Belly and chest fat is more active. It can end up in your liver, where it can raise your insulin level, blood pressure and cholesterol. It can also lead to breast and endometrial cancer.

It's not all bad news for big-bellied folks, though. Their kind of weight is a lot easier to take off.

Myth: *So what if I'm putting on weight? I'm getting older.*

Truth: You'll probably live longer if you don't gain weight as you age. "Skinny (healthy) people die at the slowest rates" is how William Castelli, M.D., medical director of the Framingham Heart Study, put it. According to his study, people who weigh anywhere from 11 to 20 percent below the average weight for people of their height have the lowest risk of death.

Myth: *I'll never lose enough weight to improve my health.*

Truth: A few pounds can make a big difference. For example, for every two pounds of excess weight you lose, your blood cholesterol drops by an average of three points. That's nothing to sneeze at.

Losing weight can help your blood pressure, too. In studies, people were able to bring their high blood pressure levels down to normal—some even went off medication—after losing as few as nine pounds. And losing nine pounds cut in half the risk of high-normal blood pressure becoming high. ("High-normal" means a diastolic pressure—the lower number—between 80 and 89.)

Myth: *A calorie is a calorie, whether it comes from a carrot or a mound of whipped cream.*

Truth: All calories are not created equal. The calories from fatty foods are more likely to make you fat than the calories from carbohydrates or protein.

Myth: *Men and women have an equally hard time losing weight.*

Truth: Men lose weight more easily than women, whether through diet or exercise. That's because men tend to be fat in their chests and bellies. And upper-body fat comes off far easier than lower-body fat. But some men and women have difficulty losing weight no matter what they do. Their genes have made them extra efficient at storing calories.

Myth: *Who needs exercise? I'm dieting.*

Truth: You need both. Most people are unable to shed more than about seven pounds through exercise alone. It's particularly tough for women. Studies show that they eat more when they're exercising regularly (men eat less). For men and women to lose serious weight, they have to eat fewer calories, particularly fat calories . . . *and* work out.

Myth: *Losing weight is a killer.*

Truth: Actually, the toughest part is keeping it off. People in supervised weight programs like those in hospitals or health clubs typically can lose 10 percent or more of their body weight. Unfortunately, they put just about all of it back on in less than five years.

But exercise—both during and after dieting—can help keep the weight off, according to Abby King and Diane Tribble of the Stanford Center for Research in Disease Prevention in Palo Alto, California. And that can get people off the yo-yo diet treadmill. There is some evidence that losing, then regaining, then re-losing weight makes it harder to

Oh, My, BMI

For years, researchers have been using the body mass index (BMI) of their subjects to help predict, among other things, how likely they are to develop certain diseases . . . or even how long they're likely to live. The Canadian Armed Forces now use the BMI instead of weight in assessing the health of their members. And the National Institutes of Health in Bethesda, Maryland, has told U.S. doctors to use it, too.

So what is this magic number?

Your BMI is your weight—in kilograms—divided by the square of your height—in meters. (Don't worry, we've converted it to pounds and inches.) Because the BMI takes into account how tall you are, it's more useful than just weight in figuring out if you're too fat.

Here's how to determine your BMI. Using the chart opposite, make a mark next to your weight (without clothes) along the left-hand scale. Then make another mark next to your height (without shoes) along the right-hand scale. Draw a line connecting the marks. The point at which the line crosses the body mass index scale down the middle of the chart is your BMI.

What Your BMI Means

Below 20: You're fine . . . if you're in good physical shape and if you aren't suffering from a disease—like cancer—that's causing you to be underweight.

take pounds off—and easier to put them back on later.

Myth: *Who cares about flabby arms? I have to get rid of these thighs.*

Truth: Exercise and diet can melt away fat, but you can't

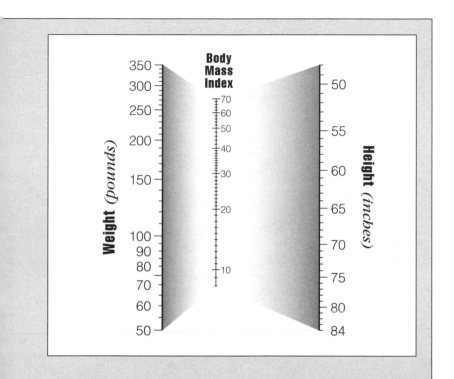

20 to 25: You're doing something right. People in this group live the longest.

26 to 30: You are overweight and have an increased risk of developing high levels of blood cholesterol, blood pressure, blood sugar and blood insulin.

Above 30: Consider yourself obese. That makes you more susceptible to diabetes, coronary heart disease, cancer and diseases of the digestive tract.

target specific areas. Women tend to lose fat from all over, while men lose it from their bellies and chests. That's just the way it happens.

—David Schardt

Shed Those Last Stubborn Pounds

Get into high gear for the race to the finish line.

Pat Jankovick laments that losing the first 30 pounds was a piece of angel food cake compared with taking off the last 10 she needs to trim to reach her goal. Teri Noble wants dearly to drop 10 pounds, but even though she eats a low-fat diet and exercises nearly every day, her scale hasn't budged for 15 years. And Carolyn Redding figures that she has peeled off the equivalent of an elephant's tonnage over the past 24 years. Too bad it was the same 10 pounds lost year after year.

What makes those last ten pounds so much harder to lose than the first ten? And once we've bombed away that weight, how do we make the blast last? We asked doctors, nutritionists and exercise physiologists: What should Pat, Teri, Carolyn and the rest of us do when we hit that seemingly insurmountable wall between us and the last ten pounds to our ideal weight?

The Dieter's Plateau

Although Pat has lost 30 pounds and improved her eating habits over the past three years, she feels as though she's stalled "in a holding pattern." Three years ago she went to a weight-loss clinic and lost 10 pounds. There she learned to watch her fats and, with continued vigilance, eventually lost 20 pounds more. Pat claims that her diet hasn't changed much since then, although she may splurge on weekends, when she dines out with her husband. She also admits to snacking on candy bars now and then. But these small dietary divergences are offset by her unwavering commitment to fitness, she says. Pat takes a 45-minute aerobics class three times a week.

Pat's predicament is a predictable one, our experts tell us. The closer we get to our ideal weight, the harder the pounds are to lose. For one thing, we tend to be highly motivated when we decide to begin a weight-loss program, so we stick to it more meticulously. But once the pounds roll off, we tend to drop our guard. Of course, an occasional dietary slip won't derail the best-laid plan. But Pat's admitted splurges are becoming habitual—a clear warning that her willpower is weakening and she's careening off course. What's worse, Pat's dietary commitment is flagging at a time when continued weight loss requires deeper caloric deficits. The diet that peeled off Pat's 30 pounds and enabled her to maintain her weight at 150 won't trim the last 10, explains James O. Hill, Ph.D., associate director of the Center for Human Nutrition at the University of Colorado Health Sciences Center in Denver.

To reach that goal, Pat will have to eat a little less or exercise a bit more. And to maintain, she'll have to continue this regimen.

What Pat needs to get herself back on track is a pat on the back, not a kick in the pants, says Diane Hanson, Ph.D., lifestyle specialist at the Pritikin Longevity Center in Santa Monica, California. Pat has "hit the wall" in her weight-loss program and probably feels that losing those last ten pounds is an insurmountable task. What she needs to do is reflect on her weight-loss accomplishments and recognize

that her goal ahead is every bit as achievable as those behind her. No matter how far Pat's come, however, she'll
continue to face those occasional urges, says Dr. Hanson.
"It's human nature. You get into a routine and then you
start to think 'How much maneuverability do I have? Is the
cheesecake going to hurt?'

"When that happens, as it has with Pat, it's time to get
yourself stirred up again and renew your commitment to
weight control," she explains. "Pat needs to reaffirm her
goals and to admit that her splurges may be undermining
her best efforts."

According to Steven B. Heymsfield, M.D., director of the
Weight Control Unit of the Obesity Research Center at
St. Luke's–Roosevelt Hospital in New York City, another
possible reason why Pat's last 10 pounds aren't loosening
their grip is that in the process of losing the first 30 pounds,
she lost muscle mass. Since muscle is metabolically active
tissue, losing muscle slows your metabolism, making the
pounds roll off more slowly. To counteract this slowdown,
Pat needs to build up calorie-burning muscle tissue, something that aerobics alone cannot do.

The best weight-loss and maintenance programs depend
on aerobics and weight-training, says James Graves, Ph.D.,
chair of the health and physical education department at
Syracuse University in New York. Aerobic workouts burn
more calories than resistance workouts, but weight-training
helps sustain a weight loss by building muscle tissue to
boost your metabolism over the long term.

Dr. Graves advises that Pat start using very light weights,
say 5 to 10 pounds for her upper body and 30 to 40
pounds for her lower body. She can start at whatever
weight she can lift comfortably for 8 to 12 repetitions. Once
12 reps becomes too easy, she can increase the weight
slightly or increase repetitions. She should aim for the types
of exercises that address the body's major muscle groups,

including arms, shoulders, chest, back, abdominals, upper legs and calves.

Stable and Stuck

Teri reads *Prevention* magazine faithfully and knows a lot about weight control. She is very fat-conscious and avoids salt. Sure, she snacks occasionally, but she sticks to low-fat, high-crunch foods like low-fat dry cereal or low-salt pretzels. Her efforts don't stop with careful eating habits: She walks a moderately paced two miles almost every day. Standing five feet four inches and holding steady at 137 pounds for the past 15 years, Teri complains, "You'd think with the way I eat and all the exercise I get, I'd look like Jane Fonda, but I can still pinch plenty of flab."

Teri has reached what Dr. Hill refers to as her settling point. This is the weight at which her body has stabilized as a result of the lifestyle habits she's settled into. Now she'll have to drive her healthy habits to a slightly higher level, he says.

Dr. Graves suggests that Teri start by intensifying her exercise program. She could easily pick up her pace, working up to a 16-minute mile. If she picks up her pace and still walks for the same amount of time, she should burn more calories, he adds.

Better yet, she'd do well to stretch a couple of her walks to three miles each week and tackle some routes with tough hills. Hill-climbing, if she maintains the same speed, can also burn more calories, says Dr. Graves. Cycling and stair-climbing could add variety to her weekly routine. Most experts agree that it doesn't matter which exercises she chooses, as long as they're convenient and fun enough that she'll do them regularly. Teri may benefit from including some weight-training, too.

Dietwise, Teri's convinced she's doing as much as she

can. Indeed, from a health standpoint, her low-fat eating habits are exemplary. But, cautions Thomas A. Wadden, Ph.D., director of the weight and eating disorders program at the University of Pennsylvania in Philadelphia, if weight loss is also a goal, the watchword is portion control. As long as Teri sticks to whole foods—fresh fruits, vegetables, grains and legumes, which are naturally high in fiber and very low in fat—her appetite should know when to call it quits. She'll feel full and satisfied on relatively few calories. The minute she sways from this fare, however, she'll have to step up her guard.

Many people fail to realize how many calories lurk in seemingly healthy foods, says Carla Wolper, a nutritionist in the Weight Control Unit of the Obesity Research Center at St. Luke's–Roosevelt Hospital. "Three popular fatteners we see in our center are Chinese food (some dishes are practically boiled in oil), those oversize bran muffins available at the corner deli (they can contain 1,000 calories each—half your daily allotment right there) and granola. A hearty bowlful can cost you 1,000 calories, not including the milk!"

Teri should read the fine print on packaged food, so she doesn't get fooled by the "lite" or "fat-free" on the labels, our experts caution.

Too often we think that just because the foods are low in fat, they're fair game for weight watchers. Teri might unwittingly consume several servings of pretzels or nonfat frozen yogurt, for example, forgetting that they're often loaded with calories.

"An article in the *New England Journal of Medicine* last year showed that people ate as much as twice what they said they were eating," says Dr. Wadden. "If Teri could prop a camera over her nose to record everything going in her mouth, she might be surprised at how much goes in.

"I'd tell Teri to keep a food diary for a week or two and

weigh and measure her portions. That way she'll see where she could cut back," he says.

More Bounce to the Ounce

Carolyn weighs the same as she did 20 years ago—about once a year. As of today, she weighs in about ten pounds more than that. But just give her a few months, and she'll slim down again! She's become a real pro at losing weight—mainly by "going on liquid diet binges" that include dietetic candy bar snacks. When she's not taking it off, she's putting it back on. And sometimes it goes on faster than it comes off—like when she travels abroad with her husband. And what about exercise? Carolyn claims she doesn't need a structured program. As a real estate agent, she gets exercise climbing in and out of cars and up and down the stairs of charming colonials and cozy Cape Cods.

Carolyn's rebounding weight problem has behavioral, not metabolic, roots, our panel of experts agrees. Although there is some evidence to the contrary, our panel rejects the theory that weight cycling—losing weight, gaining it back repeatedly—slows your metabolism and makes it harder to lose weight each time you try. As Dr. Heymsfield points out, you may temporarily add more fat than muscle when you initially regain the weight you took off, but over time, your body regains the muscle required to lug around that extra weight. So in the end, your metabolism does not slow down significantly when your weight rebounds.

To get those ten pounds off and keep them off, Carolyn would be wise to abandon her all-or-nothing approach and aim for balance.

To begin, she should wean herself from liquid fasts. These are simply short-term tactics that never, ever last, says Dr. Wadden. That's not to say that she must abandon her shakes and dietetic candy bars altogether. An occasional liquid diet drink for lunch or a low-fat frozen meal for dinner may help Carolyn keep a hold on fat and calories when mealtime circumstances threaten to take away her control.

Of course, to get Carolyn's program back on track, she needs to adjust her expectations for a slow and steady weight loss of about one pound a week. Like Teri, she should read labels, avoid both fats and sugars and stick mainly to low-fat, high-fiber grains, fruits and vegetables.

Our experts also agree that her best strategy is to expend some of her calories through exercise, because it's difficult to sustain significant calorie cuts through diet alone.

The trouble with Carolyn's occupational stair-climbing is that it doesn't provide sustained aerobic exercise, the kind that's needed to really burn calories and fat. Dr. Graves counsels that Carolyn start with fitness walking. "It's excellent exercise, it's free, and she can walk whenever she travels, too." He also suggests that Carolyn join a health club and find friends who share her goals, since social support makes it easier to stick to an exercise program.

Dr. Graves advises that Carolyn not abandon her efforts when she travels. "They can book their stays at hotels that have exercise facilities so she can keep up her efforts even when she's away from home," he says.

She can still indulge her traveling taste buds, too, he adds. Carolyn can order low-fat foods and watch her portions. Many people find that a healthy appetizer can make a very satisfying main course. "She can also take liquid diet drinks with her on trips to have for breakfast or lunch so that part of her intake is portion-controlled."

Our experts concur that the advice they gave to Pat, Teri and Carolyn could apply to anyone who wants to lose ten pounds. As Dr. Hill points out, "Most of us lose weight backward. We lose as much as we can, then try to maintain it. But the best way to get results is to lose weight slowly with permanent behavior changes that you can maintain."

Do You Really Have Ten Pounds to Lose?

Don't be duped by your bathroom scale. "Those numbers typically tell half-truths," says *Prevention* magazine's fitness advisor Wayne Westcott, Ph.D. "Your scale may tell you that you've gained 10 pounds in the past decade, when in truth you may have lost 5 pounds of muscle, then gained 15 pounds of fat. In reality, you're 20 pounds worse off."

This discrepancy can work to your advantage, too. Dr. Westcott discovered that when your exercise regimen includes weight-training as well as aerobics, your scale may show what looks like a disappointing loss of only 6 pounds after a couple of months. In fact, you may have doubled your body's improvement: You may have added 3 pounds of muscle and lost 9 pounds of fat, giving you a net improvement in body composition of 12 pounds. Your metabolism would be higher, and you could sustain your weight with more calories than you could before.

The moral of this story: Stick to a routine of resistance-training and aerobics four to six times a week—and healthy eating habits. And don't let your self-esteem rise and fall with the numbers on the scale.

Finally, when your weight stalls before you've reached your goal, be patient. "The effects of reducing fat and calories as well as exercising vary over time; don't evaluate your program too soon," cautions Dr. Hill. "Many people give up too early—the changes we've been talking about make small differences over time. Weight changes may take months or even years to show up and stabilize. Once you've begun a weight-loss program, give it at least a year to take hold for steady, long-term results."

—Jan Bresnick with Linda Rao

Easy Maintenance

There are simple ways to survive life after the diet.

Wholly underwater, you push off from the side of the pool and begin frog-kicking toward the other end. You slip effortlessly through the blue. But your body soon begs for breath, and your movements become desperate, tortured. Neck taut, lungs starved, every cell in your body screams for oxygen as you burst through the surface to swallow huge, frenzied gulps of air. Delicious.

Restrictive dieters, like swimmers, know this sensation. In essence, they hold their breath for every minute that they diet. Then, when weight loss is accomplished, say scientists at the Nutrition Research Clinic at Baylor College of Medicine in Houston, their natural inclination is to "inhale" great quantities of food, and the maintenance phase of their reduction programs becomes more challenging than even the diets themselves.

"Your body was designed to eat after dieting, just as it was designed to gasp for air after restricted breathing," explains John Foreyt, Ph.D., nutrition professor at Baylor College of Medicine, in his book *Living without Dieting*. Yet you needn't fight your natural impulse, he says: You must simply tailor it to suit your maintenance plan—in part, by gaining the proper perspective on eating and body weight.

"You must reprogram the way you think after you diet," stresses Dr. Foreyt. "The worst thing you can do is to focus solely on weight, as you did when you wanted to lose it. Weight loss is an outcome—an event—whereas maintenance is a daily process. The best way to maintain your momentum within the process is to focus on eating properly and exercising regularly."

This approach, says Dr. Foreyt, is more healthful physically and mentally than continued restrictive eating—much as breathing evenly is more comfortable than holding your breath for a time and gasping for air later.

Weight fluctuations (which may increase your risk of developing diabetes and heart disease) are less likely to occur when you're eating a balanced diet, and your life—at least as far as food goes—will probably become simpler, more even, with a more healthful focus.

Following are ten do's and don'ts that are guaranteed to facilitate weight maintenance. Some relate to perspective; others prescribe certain actions. All take a healthful, balanced approach to keeping your weight in check. Learn from them—and breathe easy.

1. DO expand your focus beyond food. "Harsh though it may sound, I put it this way—'Get a life,' " says Dr. Foreyt. "Concentrate on your well-being; build relationships with other people. A strong network of caring family and friends markedly improves your chances of keeping your weight steady. A support group can be a constant source of motivation and encouragement when you feel isolated, depressed—and primed for a binge."

2. DO continue to eat healthfully. If you followed a low-fat, high-carbohydrate regimen to pare away the pounds, stay the course. It works.

It's much more difficult for your body to store carbohydrates as body fat than to store dietary fat as body fat. As a result, your body burns more calories when it processes carbohydrates than when it processes fat—more than twice as many, in fact.

Bottom line? You can eat lots of carbohydrates and maintain your present weight and your health—the same isn't true with fat.

3. DO eat high-fiber foods every day. Fiber-rich foods, such as beans, legumes, oatmeal and sweet potatoes, are not calorically dense, meaning that you can eat a lot of them without taking in a wealth of calories. In addition, these foods take up lots of space in your stomach, so you may fill up before you consume too many calories. Finally, fiber slows the rate at which sugar enters the bloodstream, which reduces the body's insulin response. This simply means that high-fiber foods prompt the body to store less fat even as it burns more. Not bad for beans, is it?

4. DO schedule regular low-intensity workouts. Just a brisk three-mile walk burns about 300 calories. And as a calorie-burning bonus, your resting metabolic rate increases after exercise.

5. DO slow down. No matter what type of exercise you choose, the longer you do it, the more fat you'll burn. In addition, studies show that longer sessions of exercise may burn more fat than shorter, more frequent sessions. So plan to walk, bike or swim for at least 45 minutes at a time, three or more times a week. And slow down—you're sure to last longer at a comfortable pace.

6. DON'T resort to low-calorie dieting if your weight begins to creep back up. Fasting is the last thing you should do: Not only is it unpleasant, it's downright ineffective, too. When you drastically limit your food intake, your body loses muscle as well as fat, and your resting metabolic rate decreases. As a result, your body burns fewer calories at rest than it did before, and losing weight becomes exponentially more difficult.

Besides, eating too little is like holding your breath, remember? If you're like most people, you'll want to take in huge gulps of food to make up for the deficit afterward.

7. DON'T eat the same old foods you relied on to help you lose weight. Now is the time to introduce new foods into your eating plan—if only because a bored palate often spells trouble.

When you eat salad, for instance, try spinach instead of iceberg, artichoke hearts instead of mushrooms.

When you have a hankering for the latest Ben & Jerry's frozen-yogurt delight, go for it—you're in maintenance mode, after all. And when the orange roughy's on special, take some home and grill it. Treat yourself to a healthful delight every now and then; your taste buds and your psyche will thank you.

8. DON'T celebrate the new you with too much alcohol. One study concluded that alcohol may impair your body's ability to burn fat. And other research suggests that drinking alcohol with a meal may actually make you eat more.

9. DON'T make excuses for not exercising. Be creative—there are ways to work around your harried schedule. For instance, if you are traveling and plan to stay in a hotel without a gym, book a room on the 15th floor, and hike up the stairs. Take the dog on a two-mile circuit every night. And reserve an evening a week for family workouts at the YMCA.

Remember, exercise is vitally important for maintaining your ideal weight and optimal health. To quote an over-quoted yet insightful advertising campaign, "Just do it."

10. DON'T ever say never. Vows to steer clear of fudge-ripple ice cream forever will surely come back to haunt you, and you'll feel like a failure with each small indulgence. A better vow may be to savor something luscious once a week, every week. The desire is only natural, after all—like breathing. And it may stoke your motivation.

—*Linda Miller*

Part Two
Female Fat-Fighting Forces

Whose Side Is He on, Anyway?

What to do if your "better half" is inadvertently thwarting your weight-loss efforts.

In her single days, Hillary Baker could walk down Fifth Avenue and hear the sound of men's jaws smacking the pavement. She could feel their eyes—and women's, too—following her every step. And she reveled in the sensation.

Then she met Jason.

They fell in love. They got married. They became comfortable. And Hillary gained weight.

In the six months following her wedding, Hillary put on 40 pounds. More than a year later and after repeated efforts to lose the weight, she's still struggling to regain the figure that turned a thousand heads—including Jason's.

Not that Jason complains. On the contrary. "He keeps saying 'Oh, you look just fine,' " says Hillary, a 32-year-old volunteer coordinator for a Manhattan-based AIDS services center. "He insists he's still as enthralled with me as he was when I was 40 pounds lighter."

To Hillary, this notion is incomprehensible. Yet

given her husband's sunny attitude, she feels she has no incentive to take off the added weight. "If only Jason would stop trying to be nice," she says, "I could gather the support and incentive I need to try to recover my old figure. But we're just very comfortable with each other now."

Often, men like Jason truly like what they see when their mates put on weight. Of course, there are also men who don't appreciate the change but are afraid to admit it. And there are still others who fear that as their mates become slimmer, they'll also become more self-confident—and just a little too attractive.

What's with these guys, anyway?

Taking Stock

The reasons for these reactions are as numerous (and varied) as men themselves. But broad truths do apply.

If you think that the man in your life is preventing you from losing weight, you must either convince him to support you or get him out of your way. And the best way to start is by examining his actions and motives. The insight you gain will then enable you to hurdle any roadblocks your mate places in your path.

Following are descriptions of three personality types and their modi operandi. Study their patterns and search for familiar nuances. But as you do, remember that not all men undermine their mates' diets deliberately.

"Eating becomes a central feature of some couples' social lives," says Susan Olson, Ph.D., a clinical psychologist and director of psychological services at the Southeast Bariatric Nutrition Center in Scottsdale, Arizona. "And giving up those comfortable routines isn't always that easy to do."

In other words: Analyze your situation carefully—but with a charitable eye.

The Happy Camper (aka HC)

Jason is an HC. As a rule, HCs are sunny, smiling, reassuring Alan Alda types with a penchant for hand holding and quaking with fears of confrontation—not the guys you would normally think of as harboring hidden agendas.

And sometimes they don't. After all, let's not ignore the obvious: Perhaps the Happy Camper really is happy. A man may be genuinely comfortable with the apple-cheeked hausfrau his wife has become, says Maria Simonson, Sc.D., Ph.D., director of the Health, Weight and Stress Clinic at Johns Hopkins Medical Institutions in Baltimore. "Some husbands want mother images rather than conventionally beautiful and sexy wives," she explains.

But the motives of other Happy Campers may be more complicated. In fact, an HC's complacency isn't always what it seems to be, says Richard Stuart, a marriage therapist and co-author, with Barbara Jacobson, of *Weight, Sex and Marriage*. For instance, a man whose partner asks him "My thighs are huge, aren't they?" may answer in a way that is guaranteed to keep him safe from harm, says Stuart. In other words, he may lie.

Of the men with overweight wives that Stuart has interviewed in his research, 80 percent would rather their wives be thin. But when confronted with questions from their wives, such as the one posed above, many men hesitate to admit the truth for fear of alienating the women in their lives or, worse, incurring their wrath.

In all fairness to men, "Am I too fat?" questions are often posed rhetorically. And many women (and men) are actually asking for reassurance, not honesty. Still, the fact remains that women who want honest answers (and make it clear that straight shooting is what they're after) often don't get them. Instead, they get fibs or, more horrible, lines such as "So what if you're a little plump, Sugar Pie? I like you that way."

What is this Happy Camper really saying? Perhaps that he is afraid—that a thin mate might find him less dashing and debonair than he once was, that a slimmer, more attractive partner might leave him. "Implausible as it may sound, a man doesn't always want his wife or girlfriend to be attractive," says Dr. Simonson, "especially if he's insecure himself."

The Sneaky Saboteur (aka SS)

While many unsupportive men are merely noncommittal about their mates' weight loss, others are sneaky, even manipulative. They sabotage diets by placing temptation in the way: stocking the kitchen cabinets with Hershey's Chocolate Kisses, for instance—as a token of their undying affection, they insist.

This is the mark of the SS. While his approach differs from that of the Happy Camper, he probably suffers from many of the same insecurities—namely, fears of confrontation and loss. And he feels terribly threatened.

"Anytime a man tries to sabotage his mate's diet, he's really acting like a child," says Dr. Olson. The "child" is so afraid of losing his partner that he'll do anything—often quite deviously—to make sure she fails, explains Dr. Olson. He'll take her out for a romantic dinner and insist that she order the richest, most expensive dessert on the menu. Then he'll make her feel guilty if she doesn't partake of his generosity.

In a thinly disguised effort to equate food with love, he may say "I'm only trying to do something nice for you." In fact, he is trying to do the opposite—undermine his partner's attempts to lose weight, look better and feel better about herself.

The Control Freak (aka CF)

The CF is a dangerous man. Outwardly hostile, he actively opposes his partner's effort to control her weight. Like the Happy Camper and the Sneaky Saboteur, insecurity lies at the heart of the problem, but the Control Freak adds a potent and sinister element to the mix—namely, the desperate need to dominate.

Some men are hell-bent on exercising authority over the women in their lives in every way they can, says Dr. Simonson. "They become jealous if their mates do anything positive," she says. "To these men, a mate is merely a possession. She is to be only as he wants her to be. Men like this want their mates to be secondary to them in every way possible."

And there's no better way to ensure submission than to assail a woman's self-esteem, often through sarcasm and harsh criticism. For instance, a Control Freak may suggest to his mate, unkindly, that when she has tried to lose weight in the past, she has only gotten bigger, so why try again? Or he may grouse about the cost of her Weight Watchers membership, the expense of her workout tapes or the price of her special meals at Jenny Craig.

"He'll complain that she is only wasting money," says Kelly D. Brownell, Ph.D., professor of psychology at Yale University and an expert on weight loss. And he may suggest better ways to spend it—on "proper" food for him, for instance.

First cousin to the Control Freak is the Policeman. Under the guise of helping his mate achieve her weight-loss goal, he keeps track of everything she eats, often refusing to allow her to decide for herself whether one oatmeal cookie will destroy her efforts. In short, he stokes her guilt, knowing that it will work to his advantage.

"Guilt tends to produce rebellion," says Dr. Olson. "A

guilty dieter hides the cookies. And instead of eating just one, she waits until he's gone, and then she eats six.' "

Taking Charge

Undermined by the Happy Campers, Sneaky Saboteurs and Control Freaks in their lives, many women fail to lose weight. But there are plenty of other women who persevere.

Dean Reinauer of Sparta, New Jersey, is one of the latter. Several years ago, when she had just turned 28, she decided to get rid of her excess 150 pounds by spending several months at a highly successful weight-management clinic at Duke University in Durham, North Carolina. But her fiancé at the time opposed the idea.

"He didn't want me to go," she says. "He said, 'If you go, I'll be lonely.' "

But Reinauer was undeterred—even by someone who professed to love her. She went anyway, and the extra weight disappeared—along with her engagement.

Reinauer took charge of her weight and her life, and you can, too—with equally enviable results. Simply identify your goals, and take steps to achieve them. If this means addressing a dissatisfactory aspect of your relationship with your mate, don't be afraid to do so. Here's how to start.

Pay attention to what your mate does, not what he says. Remember, his actions may speak louder than his words. "He may say he loves you the way you are," says Dr. Olson, "but his body language may indicate otherwise. Maybe he's not as attentive as he once was, or maybe your love life has fallen off. If you take him at his word, you may be discouraged from dieting. But if you realize that he's sending you mixed messages, you may become more serious about controlling your eating habits."

Be blunt. If you can't muster the motivation to lose weight without your mate's involvement and support, convince him to be honest. Don't blithely accept his reassuring words. "Instead, give it to him smack between the eyes," says Dr. Simonson. "Just say 'I know you mean well, but you don't realize what you're doing when you comfort me instead of telling me what you really think.'" Lay it all on the line—and then be prepared to accept the honesty for what it is when you get it.

Spell out what you need from him. If you want him to hide the brownies, say so. If you want him to exercise with you, let him know. If you want him to keep his mouth shut, tell him that, too. Your mate can't read your mind.

"We asked women who were overweight to explain the factors that contributed to their dieting success," says Stuart. "Fifty percent attributed it to the fact that their husbands were actively involved. And the other 50 percent said they succeeded because their husbands stayed out of it altogether."

In short, there is no one right way for mates to help. It all depends on what you want, says Stuart. "The only effective approach is a frank discussion between husband and wife," he says.

Take the Control Freak by the horns. Turn the negative into a positive. Resist being drawn into a confrontation. "Say to him 'I'm sure you're just trying to help me, but it hurts me when you say these things,'" suggests Dr. Olson. "Then ask him to start making some changes in his approach. Let it be his problem, not yours."

Seek counseling if all else fails. Battles over a mate's weight are often indicative of deeper problems within a relationship, says Dr. Brownell. "A man who is giving his mate a hard time about her diet might criticize her if she wanted to learn to play the piano, too," he says. "The relationship itself is off-track, and counseling may be helpful."

Dr. Olson agrees. "In a distressed relationship, excess pounds may simply be innocent bystanders," she says. "Couples may thrash it out over an issue such as the woman's weight, but the real problem may be more substantive—such as a lack of intimacy or an imbalance of power."

Reaping Rewards

Reinauer has a new boyfriend who supports her efforts to stay slim. "I met him at my health club," she says, "and he shares my goals about myself, which we discussed as our relationship progressed.

"Once, when we were on our way to visit some of my friends," she continues, "I remembered that they had a picture of me taken at their wedding, when I was quite heavy. So I warned him that during our visit he would see a photo of me looking fat. All he said in reply was that he was very proud of me and that he couldn't believe all that I had accomplished. I couldn't believe that he was so supportive and that after so many years I finally had what I felt I deserved—what I feel every woman deserves." In three words: a supportive mate.

—Jeff Meade

The Fat Phenomenon

Give your fat cells the ol' slipperoo with this easy—and effective—alternative to dieting.

Fat cells have it hard, treated as they are to endless monologues of idle threats—promises of defacement, defeat and deletion by some do-or-die diet starting first thing in the morning. You'd think they'd hate it. But they eat it right up.

In fact, fat cells eat diets right up—literally. "New research shows that trying to starve a fat cell only improves its ability to retain fat," says Debra Waterhouse, a San Francisco nutritionist and author of *Outsmarting the Female Fat Cell*. "Diets act essentially as fitness programs for fat cells—they boost the ability of fat cells to store fat, to take in new fat and, in some cases, to increase their numbers. Although we think of diets as making us thinner, all they really do in the long run is make us fatter."

Perhaps this dynamic explains why the average American woman today weighs six pounds more than the average American woman did 30 years ago—despite the fact that women today consume, on average, about 200 fewer calories per day than women did in 1960. The difference is, women these days feed their fat cells by embarking on an average of ten diets in their lifetimes. "Diets teach fat cells to defend themselves—for reasons that cut to the heart of why we have fat cells in the first place," says Waterhouse. In a word: survival. "Fat cells evolved to keep us alive during times of famine, and they interpret a low-calorie diet as just that—famine," she explains. "Fat cells respond to famine, or calorie restriction, by holding on to the fat they already have and by becoming more aggressive at taking in new fat once the diet is over. The result is a system of fat protection that can be very difficult to crack—especially since the system becomes stronger each time we diet."

Ready for the real zinger? "Repeated dieting is so counterproductive to long-term weight control that some doctors now prescribe periods of calorie restriction followed by normal eating to help underweight people gain weight," says Waterhouse.

It's a Man's World

At least when it comes to fat, it's a man's world. Researchers looking into fat-cell physiology have found that women's fat cells are far better at developing the biochemical bullheadedness described above than men's are—hence the decidedly female focus of Waterhouse's book.

"This difference between male and female fat cells wasn't known when I first started counseling people on weight loss several years ago," says Waterhouse. "So I was confused when husbands would lose weight by the truckload while their wives would struggle to lose even a pound or two when following the same program. I thought for a while that the women were cheating."

Waterhouse was half right: She soon learned that the women, in a sense, were being cheated. Research conducted at the Cedars-Sinai Medical Center in Los Angeles showed that women are doubly damned: Not only do they possess more enzymes for storing fat, but they also have fewer enzymes burning fat. And dieting can as much as double the fat-storing enzymes and halve the fat-burning enzymes.

"This finding explains why dieting can become so self-defeating for women," says Waterhouse. "The harder we try to starve our fat cells, the more resilient they become. Men, by comparison, can diet more successfully because they don't have the enzyme profile that makes fat cells so self-protective. In addition, men are born with more muscle for burning fat through exercise."

Strike three is the female sex hormone estrogen. "Estrogen makes a woman's fat cells even more dietproof—especially in the hips, thighs and buttocks," says Waterhouse. "Studies show that men given estrogen will gain weight in these areas almost instantaneously and have a devil of a time losing it as long as they're taking estrogen."

Why? Because not only does estrogen activate and multiply fat-storing enzymes, it prompts them to multiply, too. "Estrogen is a fat cell's best friend," says Waterhouse. "And it's a dieting woman's worst enemy.

"The male fat cell developed so that it could protect one person—its male owner—from starvation during a famine," says Waterhouse. "But the female fat cell evolved so that it could protect two—its female owner and her developing fetus. The better a woman's fat-storing capability, the greater the chances that she—and the entire species—will survive. In fact, if the female fat cell hadn't evolved to be so cantankerous, we might not be here today."

Plan for Patience

The primary focus of diet research today is whether these primal forces can be altered or shaped to our liking. According to Waterhouse, they can.

"The key to permanent weight loss is to resist trying to bully your body chemistry through crash diets and grueling exercise routines," she says. "Instead, try to conquer it with kindness. Proceed so slowly and cautiously that your fat cells don't get shocked into mounting their systems of self-defense."

Permanent weight loss, after all, requires major changes: It demands that a woman alter her body's biochemical infrastructure so that she produces fewer enzymes for storing fat and more for burning it. "And this takes time," says Waterhouse. "The mistake so many women make is trying to rush the process—they end up strengthening the very systems they're trying to weaken."

Bottom line: no more diet sodas for breakfast, carrot sticks for lunch and dinners from plastic pouches. No more 2½-hour fitness routines that leave you swimming in sweat. No more miracle powders, grapefruits or sweat suits. "Heroic displays of willpower don't lead to permanent weight loss," says Waterhouse. "Funny as it sounds, weight-loss plans are doomed by the degree to which they become a struggle."

Ease is the key. To that end, Waterhouse has put together the following six-step plan for just the sort of long-term, fat-cell-foiling, body-chemistry makeover that she promises will result in permanent weight loss. The program, which relies on research conducted at several institutions including the Cedars-Sinai Medical Center and Johns Hopkins University in Baltimore, currently boasts a long-term (five-year) success rate that exceeds that of most commercial weight-loss programs by about tenfold.

"But don't take it up like a life raft," cautions Waterhouse. "Remember to go slowly and respect your body's right to feel properly nourished. If you incorporate just one of these six strategies into your lifestyle every two weeks or so, you'll achieve success."

Step 1: Exercise Comfortably

That's right: Work out in moderation. "Exercise is the single most important step a woman can take to alter her fat-storing chemistry," says Waterhouse. "But just as with dieting, exercising beyond your comfort level panics your fat cells and causes them to cling to the very fat you want them to release. Once you slip into oxygen debt—meaning that you're gasping for breath—your muscles use glycogen, which is a carbohydrate, for fuel instead of fat."

Walking at a pace that prompts you to breathe deeply and rhythmically without gasping is ideal for fat burning, although any activity that employs major muscle groups is excellent. Try cycling, swimming, running, rowing, stair-climbing, in-line skating or continuous aerobics, and gradually work up to exercising for 45 minutes without stopping at least three times a week, Waterhouse says. (Four or five sessions would be even better.) "Studies show that optimal fat utilization can take as long as 30 minutes to kick into gear," says Waterhouse. "So if you exercise for 45 minutes, you'll burn fat best during the final 15."

And don't be afraid to add variety to your routine. According to Waterhouse, mastering an assortment of activities that work different muscle groups stimulates fat burning even more than sticking with one activity. "By all means, spread the fat-burning wealth around," she says. "Walk one day, cycle another and tackle a third activity, such as swimming or strength-training, that works the muscles in your shoulders and arms. The more muscles you whip into shape, the better your body will become at burning fat."

Why? Because muscle tissue burns more calories at rest than fat tissue. "Adding muscle not only increases the calories you burn as you exercise," says Waterhouse, "but also boosts the calories you burn while you're asleep. Now that's a weight-control advantage that shouldn't be missed!"

Step 2: Eat Heartily

Exercise is the single most effective way to get your fat cells to release their fat instead of storing it—but only if you eat properly as part of your fitness regimen. If you restrict your eating, your fat cells will remain in their fat-protecting posture, and your muscles will be forced to supply the energy for your workouts. Consequently, you'll diminish the very muscle you're trying to build!

"This is difficult for many women to believe," says Waterhouse, "and I understand why. It seems logical that dieting should make exercise burn more fat rather than less, but it doesn't. Dieting while exercising forces muscles to consume themselves if necessary for the energy they need. Strange as it sounds, you must give your muscles the calories they need to burn fat if you want them to do so."

Waterhouse doesn't recommend stuffing yourself indiscriminately, but she does suggest that you eat in response to your body's natural hunger signals. For most women, this means consuming between 1,400 and 2,400 calories a day.

Step 3: Resist Overeating

This may sound obvious, but it's not. "Most of us overeat without even realizing it," says Waterhouse. "We eat to the point of feeling full rather than simply satisfied. And we eat when we're not really hungry. Or we starve and then stuff ourselves. All of these patterns qualify as overeating, and fat cells are quick to capitalize on them. Fat cells respond to overindulging in much the same way they do to undereating—they throw themselves into a fat-storing frenzy."

Striking a balance is crucial. "The only way to keep your fat cells from becoming hyperactive is to take in the number of calories your body needs to function—no more, no less," says Waterhouse.

The first step in gaining awareness of your eating patterns is to identify the reasons you're eating, perhaps by keeping a food diary. "Eating for emotional reasons—because you're bored, stressed, angry or depressed—is very fattening," says Waterhouse, "mostly because it has very little to do with what your body actually requires. What's more, eating doesn't address the problem, so it becomes a symptom rather than a cure."

The second step is easier: Simply pay attention to your feelings of fullness when you eat—and stop just as you're beginning to feel satisfied.

Step 4: Shrink and Multiply Your Meals

Forget logic—weight loss involves nonlinear thinking. Here's why: One meal of 2,000 calories is more fattening than two meals of 1,000, and two meals of 1,000 calories are more fattening than four of 500.

"The math seems strange until you think about it," says Waterhouse. "If you eat more calories than your body can burn in a few hours, the rest will be stored as fat." This is why women who do most of their eating in one or two meals a day make a costly mistake. "They think they're cutting calories," says Waterhouse, "but proportionately, more of the calories they're eating turn to fat."

The key to weight control, then, is to limit excess calories, which wander around in the bloodstream and eventually get picked up by fat cells. And the only way to pull this off is to eat smaller meals at more frequent intervals.

"Divide the amount of food you're currently eating into four, five or six meals," suggests Waterhouse. "Even if you wind up eating slightly more calories than you're accustomed to, they'll be more evenly distributed throughout the day and hence less fattening."

Step 5: Limit Nighttime Eating

Padlock the fridge after about 7:00 P.M., because fat cells do their best work after dark. "Calories that would be used productively by the body if they were eaten during the day get stored as fat if they're eaten in the evening," says Waterhouse. "There's little physical demand on the body at night and little competition for the calories by the body's other systems."

To illustrate the "eat light at night" rule, Waterhouse cites a physician who became legendary in the 1930s for helping people lose weight based on a single request—that his clients eat dinner no later than 5:00 P.M.

"Modern-day work schedules have rendered this goal impractical for most people," Waterhouse admits. "But we can all try to eat a small dinner as early as possible and limit our nighttime snacking." If you find that this strategy leaves you hungry, you may be eating too little during the day.

Step 6: Eat Less Fat

You were waiting for this one, weren't you?

"I'm not suggesting you become a fat phobe and limit yourself to fruits and vegetables," says Waterhouse. "I only advise that you cut back on fatty cuts of meat, fried foods, full-fat dairy products, eggs, cheese, fatty salad dressing and sauces and gravies made with cream, butter or high-fat meat."

Fat is more than twice as dense with calories as protein or carbohydrates. What's more, fat is first in line for storage by fat cells because it qualifies as fat already. "Proteins and carbohydrates need to go through considerable chemical conversions before fat cells can accept them," says Waterhouse. "Not so with dietary fats. They're in a form that fat cells can welcome the minute they enter the bloodstream."

Given this scenario, Waterhouse formulated a three-to-one rule for limiting the fat in your diet to no more than 25 percent of the total number of calories you consume: "Every time you eat a food that is high in fat, simply balance it with three others that are low in fat," she says. "For instance, you can compensate for a dinner that includes fried chicken by eating a plain baked potato, a steamed vegetable and a piece of fresh fruit along with it."

How do you know which foods are high in fat and which are low? Read food labels, suggests Waterhouse. "If a food contains more than 2.5 grams of fat per 100-calorie serving, it derives more than 25 percent of its calories from fat."

—Porter Shimer

Part Three

A Guy's Guide to Leanness

Live Like a Bachelor, Eat Like a Man

How a single guy can get decent nutrition without actually entering a kitchen.

Nothing, they say, changes a man like marriage. What is a useful telltale signal of marriage's impact? Try food. You can tell the difference right away between a married man and a bachelor by the questions each asks about food. For example, a married man is likely to ask something like this: "Hey, honey, what's for dinner?"

A bachelor question goes something like this: "Why is it we can put a man on the moon but we can't solve the twin dilemmas of diet and laundry by making an edible gym sock that, when lightly microwaved, tastes like pizza?"

Every bachelor has a unique tale of heartbreak and anguish, of loneliness and despair, of cheap pick-up lines and memorable nights with beauty queens. But all bachelors have one thing in common: They all have to eat.

The bad news is, sometimes you have to eat alone. The good news is, you can live like a bachelor and still eat like a man—provided you're willing to pick up a few general principles and apply them to single-guy eats.

Statistics show single guys croak early, while married men live long and prosper. Food probably has something to do with that. The marital board is lush and regular and usually has something green on it. In a bachelor fridge, only the cheese is green. You could die eating bachelor grub. So here, as an appetizer, are five simple rules for surviving the nutritional potholes on the solitary road, followed by a bite-by-bite exploration of the principal bachelor food groups.

These may at first seem elementary, Watson, but if you're like most bachelors, you haven't been paying much attention to them anyway, so they bear repeating.

1. Mom's Law. For most of us, women have been the kitchen kops, working the dietary beat since day one. For example, there's the Universal Principle of the Golden Nutritional Mean, also known as Mom's Law. Mom's Law says "Eat three squares a day." No way? No time? Then graze. Eat small portions several times a day. Mom probably once told you this was a bad idea, but she's changed her mind. Now it's okay, as long as you make your snacks something remotely healthy: a piece of fruit, a bagel, air-popped popcorn or a bag of pretzels. The idea here is never to go without eating for longer than five hours. Brain drain and fatigue lie that way.

Mom's Law also has a predictable corollary: "Don't skip breakfast." Eat a slice of toast with a glass of fruit juice, a bowl of cereal or three pancakes from any fast-food chain. (The syrup's okay, but skip the butter.) Something in the morning jump-starts the system and helps you manage your eating throughout the day.

2. Svelteness by the Numbers. For every 3,500 calories you eat beyond what your body burns, you'll gain a pound. For every 3,500-calorie deficit, you lose a pound.

For instance, the rough requirement for most average-size men is 2,500 calories a day. Let's say you're an average guy, and let's say part of your daily diet is two Kit Kat bars. That's 460 calories a day of Kit Kat nutrition. Skip those bars, and you're down to around 2,000 calories a day. If you suck up only 2,000 calories every day, you'll lose about a pound a week on average. Exercise is excellent, of course, and helps your body burn up, rather than store, calories. But exercise alone won't do it. You must reduce your calorie intake, too.

3. The Iron Law of Fat. Avoid it when you can. There. Read the package label or the handouts many restaurants provide. Normally, the amount of fat is given in grams per serving. Each gram of fat provides 9 calories. Multiply the number of grams by 9. Divide that number by the total number of calories in a serving. What you get is the percentage of calories from fat. Think hard about anything that gets 30 percent or more of its total calories from fat. For example, four frozen fish sticks have 12 grams of fat and 280 calories, which may not look too bad. But 12 times 9 divided by 280 reveals that 39 percent of the calories come from fat. Bad.

If this is too much math for you, think of it this way: Try to keep it under three grams of fat per 100 calories.

4. The Equally Iron Law of Salt. Don't add salt to anything. Food preparers habitually oversalt. The National Academy of Sciences suggests no more than 2,400 milligrams of sodium a day, or about a teaspoon of salt. Remember that number: 2,400. Look at the food labels. Some frozen chicken entrées, for example, contain up to 1,000 milligrams, and some frozen chicken complete dinners exceed 2,000. That's a pillar of salt in anybody's book, especially when you consider salt's link to life-shortening high blood pressure.

5. The Cholesterol Controversy. A little while ago, bad-boy foods like whole eggs, which contain buck-naked cholesterol, were seen as heart-stoppers. Eat an egg and die, the science boys said.

They were sort of right: It's a good idea to eat less rather than more. But the new rule says not to eliminate cholesterol completely unless there's a medical reason to do so. The most recent recommendation is to top out at about 300 milligrams of cholesterol a day. A fast-food scrambled egg platter can give you that or more; you wouldn't want to do too many of those.

That's all the law you need. Now for some science.

Nutritionists love charts showing the basic food groups, with nice little illustrations in case you've forgotten what a leafy vegetable looks like. You should eat a little dairy, lots of fruits and vegetables, a little less meat and a little more fish and chicken and lots more grains and beans.

But we know that for single men, real life isn't so neat. To the extent that a busy man thinks at all about nutrition's little laws, he probably sees the world of chow organized around the BFGs, or bachelor food groups.

The Drive-Thru Food Group

This group includes everything you get from fast-food chains, roach coaches, vending machines and lots of restaurants, including the cafeteria at work.

If you're a man on the move, you're at a disadvantage, dietwise, and food preparers can shovel just about anything they want into you. But enough of you have spoken up that chains and restaurants are now calling attention to low-fat or low-calorie specials and vegetarian offerings. Not all are as lean as they would have you believe. But check these items out.

• Carl's Jr. Le Potato gets only 3 percent of its calories from fat and contains no cholesterol and a mere 60 milligrams of sodium.

• McDonald's McLean Deluxe sandwich gets 28 percent of its calories from fat and delivers slightly more than 650 milligrams of sodium.

• Hardee's grilled chicken breast sandwich gets 26 percent of its calories from fat and contains acceptable levels of sodium and cholesterol. In general, chicken sandwiches are healthy, provided they aren't made from big slabs of fried chicken.

• Long John Silver's baked fish with lemon crumbs gets a scant 17 percent of its calories from fat and has 680 milligrams of sodium.

• El Pollo Loco's flame-broiled chicken salad gets 16 percent of its calories from fat and contains only 375 milligrams of sodium.

• In fact, salads, generally, are a good idea. You know that. But the only way to keep them good, friend, is to keep your paws away from the dressings. Exceptions: a drop or two of oil with all the vinegar you want; any of the Kraft Free dressings, which have no fat at all; or any other low-fat dressings that get less than 30 percent of their calories from fat.

Meanwhile, avoid these.

• Breakfast sausage platters—just about anyone's: You're looking at 60 percent fat and 1,000 milligrams of sodium, minimum.

• Tricky salads: Chef and taco salads can get 40 to 60 percent of their calories from fat. And sodium for both can top 1,000 milligrams.

• Tricky sandwiches: Croissant sandwiches with egg and bacon or cheese get 60 percent or more of their calories from fat.

- Burgers: Sorry, but the truth is, McDonald's is about the only place with a burger that gets less than 30 percent of its calories from fat. And almost everything burgerlike contains from a third to half of all the salt you should be consuming in an entire day—and that's before you start salting it.
- Avoid deep-fried fish. It's likely to be fattier than a burger.

Sometimes the adjectives are a giveaway: Stay away from anything described as creamed or creamy, au gratin or buttery. There are alternatives, fortunately. Look for these words: grilled, charbroiled, flame-broiled, baked, roasted, boiled or in its own sauce (or juice).

The Food That Drives to You Group

- Pizza: What sort of shameless food would come knocking at your front door? If you're having it brought in, it's probably pizza. Pizza's not necessarily awful food, but it's hardly perfect, either. A pizza secret: Simpler is better. Cut down on the cheese. If you can hold the pepperoni, do so. Vegetables are fine.

  A slice of basic cheese pizza gets 28 percent of its calories from fat and contains about 700 milligrams of sodium. Not bad, right? But the same pizza with extra cheese and pepperoni can double the fat and push sodium over 1,000 milligrams. That's about how it runs across the big pizza board.
- Chicken: Avoid fried chicken. Period.
- Wok on wheels: One of the hipper trends in home delivery is Oriental foods, mostly Chinese and Thai. Many of these dishes are high in oil and sodium. To cut down on both, always get steamed rice instead of fried. Avoid egg rolls, dumplings and higher-fat dishes, such as those using

pork, and head toward the chicken end of the menu, or better yet, choose from the vegetable list—get it steamed.

The Supermarket Food Group

The Supermarket Food Group is composed of two classes: (1) food you buy to eat and (2) food you feel you have to buy when you're really just there to meet girls. The frozen-food department at the supermarket is the singles bar of the microwaving singles set. Since you have to buy something to provide decent cover, you need to heed the rules of smart shopping. In general:

- Again, simpler is better. For example, frozen chicken pot pies are almost always higher in everything you don't want than roasted chicken entrées.
- Read the fine print. Even if an item is low in, say, calories, it might be a killer when it comes to sodium or fat. Also, don't get caught believing that "lower-fat" is synonymous with "low-fat." Lower just means it has less than it used to, which may have been a lot.
- Cups of noodles may have only 200 to 300 calories but can top 40 percent in calories from fat and are loaded with salt.
- Some brands of "light" batter fish get more than half of their calories from fat, which is actually more than some regular fish fillets or fish sticks.
- Vienna sausages are out of the question. The tiny weenies are above 80 percent in calories from fat and run as high as 750 milligrams of sodium per serving.

It's not entirely hopeless. There are a number of frozen dishes that will do when the microwave is all you have time for. All the entrées and dinners below meet our low-fat standard. Just be sure to fit their sodium contribution into what you're getting the rest of the day.

• Healthy Choice roasted turkey and mushrooms in gravy gets 14 percent of its 200 calories from fat and has 380 milligrams of sodium.

• Weight Watchers new shrimp marinara with linguine has only 150 calories and less than a gram of fat. It has 390 milligrams of sodium.

• Le Menu Healthy golden glazed chicken gets only 8 percent of its 330 calories from fat and has 420 milligrams of sodium.

• Budget Gourmet Light and Healthy teriyaki beef has 270 calories, six grams of fat and 520 milligrams of sodium.

• Stouffer's Lean Cuisine three-cheese French bread pizza gets 27 percent of its 330 calories from fat and has 350 milligrams of sodium.

The Do-It-Yourself Food Group

This group consists of the stuff you buy and actually cook for yourself. So we're talking spaghetti here, right? Right. Spaghetti contains almost no fat and won't salt your innards for you. Tomato spaghetti sauce is ambrosia for the health-conscious bachelor. But if you want to get downright Italo-cool, simply heat a half-teaspoon of olive oil and mix in any or all of these: a clove of minced garlic, a handful of sunflower seeds, some chopped parsley, a sliced Japanese eggplant or Italian squash, some sun-dried tomatoes, red pepper flakes or capers. Toss with pasta, and you have a fine meal.

See, single guys need style, in the kitchen as much as elsewhere, and nothing makes you feel more like the master of your own destiny than going out to the supermarket, stalking some real food, bagging it at the checkout and taking it back to the den for a little prep.

For instance, buy some boneless chicken breasts. Because they're also skinless, nearly all the fat has been pulled off for you. Put the breasts in a pan with some canned low-sodium chicken stock and a few slices of garlic. Cover and simmer until the chicken's done. Zap, a meal.

The Danger Food Group

• Supermarket roulette: Most types of coleslaw, hot dogs and sausages, like pepperoni, chorizo and liverwurst, are sky-high in fat, while soufflés, whole eggs, ice cream, custard and even shrimp are disproportionately high in cholesterol.

The vile and dreaded salt monsters come cleverly disguised as dill pickles, canned soups, specialty items like onion or garlic salt, cheese, salted nuts, olives and soy, barbecue and curry sauces, not to mention innocent-seeming cottage cheese. Some lunch meats are more than 50 percent fat and contain 2,000 milligrams of sodium per serving. Stick to chicken, turkey and seafoods, such as water-packed tuna. Just be sure to hold the mayo and the Russian dressing.

• Alcohol: Liquid idiot is high in calories and has practically nothing else of any value except the ability to make you forget your own true love and the nation's deficit. But you knew that already, didn't you?

That's the nutrition part. But are we not men? Death will not follow instantaneously upon ingestion of moderate quantities of any of the above; nor will occasional bacheloresque forays into nutritional vice wreck your constitution or immediately balloon you into obesity. Destroying a man's body takes time. Which also means that with a little effort, and sense, you can maintain your peace of mind and body weight and help yourself avoid bodily malfunction.

Even if you're a bachelor.

—Bruce Henstell

Another Side of Beef

Don't have a cow, but the old-fashioned steak houses are back. Are they a nutritional nightmare or a harmless indulgence?

It's a no-frills steak house with only three entrées on the menu—Little Dogie (8 ounces), Cattleman's Dream (16 ounces) and Big Bull (32 ounces). Because I haven't eaten all day and an uncle is picking up the tab, I do what many guys would do. Fifteen minutes of expert charbroiling later, my Big Bull arrives sizzling on a metal platter. The waitress hands me what looks like a bowie knife and a bib, then wishes me good luck with Ferdinand.

I consider myself a relatively active, health-conscious guy, yet there I was, chowing down on a hunk of meat the size of my face. And I wasn't alone. All around me, dozens of guys were satiating their carnivorous instincts with abandon. It was as though words like "cholesterol" and "coronary" were a forgotten segment of the lexicon. Isn't meat poison?

Though I didn't know it at the time, I was part of a growing trend. All over the country, upscale steak houses are sprouting up, and the cattle industry is rejoicing. Over 100 million more orders of beef were served up in restaurants in '93 than in '92, and even

'92 was a banner year. Why the sudden change in attitude after years of condemning cows for everything from heart disease to the greenhouse effect? Maybe it's a backlash to the weight-watching '80s. The more important question is, are we all headed for heart attacks, or is the occasional trip to Sirloin City an acceptable part of healthy living?

Most of the experts agree that although eating too much meat is a mistake, so, too, is looking at it as poison. "You shouldn't focus on single food groups as if they were 'good' or 'bad,'" says C. Wayne Callaway, M.D., clinical nutritionist at George Washington University Medical Center in Washington, D.C. "Restricting red meat in isolation of the total diet is an irrational thing to do."

"The main issue is how much saturated fat is in your diet, not where it comes from," says John C. LaRosa, M.D., former chairperson of the nutrition committee and task force on cholesterol of the American Heart Association. Saturated fat is a major culprit in heart disease, since it depresses the liver's ability to filter cholesterol out of the bloodstream. Most dairy products contain plenty of saturated fat. It's also found to a lesser extent in certain plant foods, such as avocados, Brazil nuts and coconuts. Palm oil, a vegetable product, contains significantly more saturated fat than even lard. But how much palm oil do you guzzle on a given day? "If you look at sources of saturated fat in the American diet," says Dr. LaRosa, "the single most common food source is beef, because it is such a widely consumed food."

The drawbacks of consuming regular Big Bull quantities of beef are well-known. In a study of 26,473 Seventh-Day Adventists (who rarely drink and do not smoke), men who ate beef at least three times a week had more than twice the risk of developing fatal heart disease as those whose diets were beef-free.

Another rap against cattle roundups is the high dose of iron they deliver. Depending on the cut, three ounces of cooked beef provides from 20 to 30 percent of the recommended daily amount. The male body stores and recycles iron quite efficiently and may easily overload. In fact, in one Finnish study, having high levels of iron in the blood ranked second only to cigarette smoking as a risk factor for male heart disease. While there's debate over the report—William Castelli, M.D., medical director of the Framingham Heart Study, told us the Finnish report needs to be substantiated by a larger study before we leap to conclusions—the findings tend to argue for moderation.

Still another particularly male problem is the apparent link between some of the fatty acids red meat contains and prostate cancer. As part of the ongoing Physicians' Health Study, Harvard researchers found that men who dined on beef, pork or lamb at least 5 times a week were 2.5 times more likely to develop prostate cancer than those who dined on the same 3 times a month or less.

On the other hand, the beef industry has been raising leaner cattle. Compared with those of ten years ago, today's steaks are nearly 30 percent leaner; burgers are 10 percent leaner. "A person can easily consume six or seven ounces of lean meat per day and stay within recommended fat limits," says Mary Bielamowicz, R.D., Ph.D., a nutrition specialist at Texas A & M University in College Station.

Easily? For her, maybe. The centerpiece of this hypothetical beef-fest is a less-than-majestic serving—usually described as a portion about the size of two decks of cards. The medical endorsement for eating even this much daily also presupposes that one is holding the line on other sources of saturated fat. Like butter. Like Häagen-Dazs.

If you want to keep eating meat, leading researchers in both food science and heart disease suggest the following.

Get good grades. The U.S. Department of Agriculture grades beef based on fat marbling. Prime contains the most fat. Next is Choice, and lowest is Select. How much fat each

Beefing about Fat

All beef is not created equal. Fat and calorie values vary considerably from cut to cut. Three ounces of ground beef, for example, has three times as much fat as the same size portion of beef top round and over 50 additional calories.

The following table ranks various cuts of beef in order of increasing fattiness. Using this table, you can plan a diet that derives less than 30 percent of calories from fat, as recommended by the American Heart Association.

Cut	Calories from fat (%)	Fat (g)	Calories
Top round steak	25	4.2	153
Eye round roast	26	4.2	143
Shank cross cut	28	5.4	171
Tip round steak	34	5.9	157
Arm pot roast	35	7.1	184
Bottom round roast	35	7.0	178
Top loin steak	41	8.0	176
Filet mignon	43	8.5	179
Flank steak	44	8.6	176
T-bone steak	44	8.8	182
Porterhouse steak	45	9.2	185
Blade roast	47	11.1	213
Brisket	47	10.9	206
Rib eye steak	47	10.0	191
Ground beef	57	13.9	218

grade contains depends upon the cut. For example, a Prime tenderloin steak gets 48 percent of its calories from fat. The same steak rated Choice gets about 44 percent of its calories from fat, and a Select steak, 39 percent.

Catch up on your reading. Check the table on the opposite page to find the fat content of various cuts of beef. Lean cuts such as top round steak have about one-third the fat of ground beef.

Watch the language. Look for the words "round" or "loin" when shopping for beef and the words "loin" or "leg" when purchasing pork. Say "white meat" when ordering chicken. All these words mean lower fat content.

Make the cut. Trim off visible fat before cooking. When meat is cooked with external fat on it, a small amount migrates to the lean tissue. Avoid eating the skin on chicken and other forms of poultry.

Don't add fat to the fire. That means don't fry meat in oil or broil your filet mignon with a ring of bacon.

Rack it up. Roast, bake or barbecue meat on a rack so that excess fat can drip away.

Finally, the experts do offer one kind indulgence. They say you can go on the occasional meat-eating bacchanalia without undermining your good health, as long as you're very good about avoiding fat most of the time. "There have been studies on how often you can binge without really changing your cholesterol level," says Dr. LaRosa. "It turns out you can eat anything you want once a week, and it won't really matter.

"The trouble is," Dr. LaRosa says, "in the United States, 'every once in a while' does not exist. We think that if it's okay once a week, why not two or three times a week? Then pretty soon it's every night." A point well taken. Next time I visit that char house, I'll make mine the Little Dogie.

—Jim Thornton

Fuel Injection

30 quick and easy ways to power up your favorite foods.

It's safe to say that the curve representing modern man's meal-preparation time has grown exceedingly short. Where our forefathers were willing to track a caribou for days in order to get a decent steak, now waiting even 20 minutes for a pizza delivery tries our patience.

With time at such a premium, nutrition often suffers. We know that a steady diet of the quick and the packaged jams our bodies with too much fat, salt and cholesterol, but perhaps more important is what these meals aren't doing. Unplanned meals eaten on the run tend to be low in the vitamins that energize us, keep our immune systems strong and charge up our brains. The more time-pressed a man is, the more he needs to be sure that his diet is top-notch. "Whether you're a linebacker or a guy in the front office, you have to put the right fuel in your engine," says Dean Kleinschmidt, head athletic trainer for the New Orleans Saints.

Usually, it doesn't take any more time to make and eat a nutritious meal than a poor one. Below are 30 no-brains-necessary ways to power up your favorite foods without sacrificing taste—or time. We'll start with a quick explanation of the key ingredients of good nutrition, but if you already know this stuff, skip right ahead to the meals.

Complex carbohydrates. Foods like pastas, breads, cereals, beans, vegetables and fruits are loaded with these. Carbohydrates are a powerful fuel whose calories pump up your energy level, not your waistline.

Fiber. Found in fruits, vegetables, beans and grains, fiber goes through your system like a sponge, absorbing cholesterol and clearing it away. Studies suggest a high-fiber diet also helps prevent colon cancer and may help control blood sugar levels in people with adult-onset diabetes.

Antioxidants. Oxidation, the same chemical reaction that causes sliced apples to turn brown, also takes place in our bodies and has been linked to cancer, heart disease and the aging process. *Anti*oxidants, like vitamins C and E and beta-carotene, prevent oxygen particles from doing their damage within the body. Top sources of antioxidants are orange juice, red bell peppers, strawberries and broccoli for vitamin C; wheat germ, olive oil and safflower oil for vitamin E; and carrots, spinach, sweet potatoes and cantaloupe for beta-carotene.

Calcium. This building block of strong teeth and bones can help ward off osteoporosis (men make up 20 percent of all cases), lower blood pressure, prevent kidney stones and reduce LDL (low-density lipoprotein) cholesterol, the bad kind. Besides skim milk, fortified orange juice, yogurt, salmon and green leafy vegetables are sources of calcium.

Potassium. This mineral may lower blood pressure and prevent heart attacks and strokes. Good sources are potatoes, raisins, orange juice and bananas.

B vitamins. Studies show that some of the B's play important roles in brain function and memory. And B_6 is believed to be important for maintaining a strong immune system. You'll get one or more of the B vitamins from pastas, sunflower seeds, skim milk, chicken breast, bananas, potatoes, clams or chick-peas.

Magnesium. Deficiencies in magnesium may put you at increased risk of heart disease, kidney stones and gallstones. You'll get magnesium from sunflower seeds, wheat germ, spinach and almonds.

Zinc. This mineral, found in wheat germ, oysters and beef, helps your immune system fight off viruses, and it's a key ingredient in the production of healthy sperm.

30 Ways to Give Your Food a Lift

1. Energize bottled spaghetti sauce with carbohydrate-rich squash, beans, peas, broccoli and onion. Chop the vegetables, zap them in the microwave for 20 or 30 seconds and throw them right in the sauce.

2. Don't like big chunks of vegetables in your sauce? You can get almost double the daily recommended levels of beta-carotene, plus 4.6 grams of fiber, by grating two carrots finely and mixing them in. You won't even know they're there.

3. Get 500 percent of the Recommended Dietary Allowance (RDA) of zinc, 800 percent of the RDA of vitamin B_{12}, some magnesium and heart-healthy fish oil by adding just six medium oysters to your marinara sauce.

4. Boost dietary fiber in spaghetti 6.4 grams by substituting whole-wheat pasta for the low-fiber white-flour kind.

5. Raise the fiber and carbohydrate content of your chili—and lower the fat—by cutting the amount of beef you normally use in half and substituting the same amount of red kidney beans. Trim fat in chili even further by substituting ground turkey or chicken breast for the beef.

6. Add vitamin C, beta-carotene and B vitamins to your lasagna by following this quick recipe from *What's Cooking at the Cooper Clinic,* a cookbook from the Dallas fitness

center's nutrition department. You can make the entire meal in less than an hour. One helping delivers 3 grams of fiber, 33 grams of carbohydrates, 22 grams of protein and a lot less fat than traditional lasagna. Preheat the oven to 375°. Spray the bottom of a 9 × 12-inch casserole dish with cooking spray. Pour a 28-ounce jar of spaghetti sauce in a bowl and mix in 1 cup of water. In another bowl, combine 16 ounces of low-fat cottage cheese and ¼ cup of part-skim grated mozzarella cheese, ¼ cup of fat-free egg substitute, 1 teaspoon of garlic powder and ¼ teaspoon of ground black pepper.

To construct the lasagna: Coat the bottom of the dish with sauce, then place a layer of uncooked lasagna noodles on top. Cover the noodles with another layer of sauce, then spoon the cheese mixture over the sauce. Next, add a layer of cooked and drained spinach and/or sliced raw zucchini. Cover the vegetables with a layer of noodles, then sauce, then cheese mixture. Finally, add the remaining sauce, making sure that the noodles are completely covered. Bake uncovered for 50 minutes. Sprinkle some grated mozzarella cheese over the lasagna during the last 15 minutes of baking.

7. Make a high-energy omelette by adding canned sliced potatoes for more carbohydrate power. Start by mixing two egg whites with two whole eggs to limit the cholesterol. Mix the eggs with sliced mushrooms, red and green bell peppers, onions, canned potatoes (chopped) and a shot of skim milk, which will add calcium and make the eggs fluffy. You can also take the cholesterol-cutting one step further by using fat- and cholesterol-free egg substitutes. You'll find them in the dairy or frozen-food case at the supermarket.

8. Make a leaner meat stew by substituting chicken for beef. Boost the carbohydrate level by packing in plenty of potatoes, rice or pasta. Here's an easy, high-powered recipe that's delicious.

Get a pound of boneless chicken breast, two cans of

low-fat, reduced-salt chicken broth and a ten-ounce package of mixed frozen vegetables. Cut the chicken into chunks. Dump the chicken, vegetables and broth into a pot. Add a chopped clove of garlic and cook over medium heat about 15 minutes, or until the chicken is done. Then, ladle out the chicken and vegetables and place them on a plate. Put one cup of rice, one cup of macaroni or pasta shells or one large potato (cubed) in the broth. Bring to a boil, then reduce heat and allow to cook for 10 minutes. Dump the chicken and vegetables back in the pot and simmer for 5 more minutes.

9. Pack your pizza with vitamins by topping the pie with any of the following: broccoli, green and red peppers, eggplant, mushrooms, cauliflower and tomato slices. Remember, too, that any pizza-improvement project depends as much on what you take off as on what you add on. So before you pile on the vegetables, delete the pepperoni for a savings of 7.6 grams of fat in just two slices. Also, next time you're ordering a pie, ask them to use half the cheese they normally do.

10. Add some muscle to macaroni and cheese by sprinkling some crunchy wheat germ on top before baking. One-quarter cup of wheat germ offers 50 percent of the RDA of folate, a B vitamin important to the production of red blood cells, and 40 percent of the RDA for vitamin E. You'll also want to trim the fat by substituting a low-fat sharp Cheddar for the regular kind. One to try: Kraft Light Naturals Sharp Cheddar Reduced-Fat Cheese. The adventurous eater who wants more fiber and carbohydrates can also add a package of mixed frozen vegetables or a can of white kidney beans or great Northern beans.

11. Make a huge bowl of antioxidant-rich fruit salad and keep it in your refrigerator so you can dip into it all week. Combine in a bowl the following:

1 pink grapefruit, peeled and sectioned
1 large navel orange, peeled and sectioned

1 mango, sliced
1 cup cantaloupe chunks
1 cup honeydew chunks
1 cup strawberry halves
½ cup raspberries or other berries
In a smaller bowl, mix together:
½ cup nonfat vanilla yogurt
2 tablespoons orange juice
1 tablespoon lime juice

Pour the yogurt topping over the fruit and mix well. Spoon onto a plate and sprinkle with sunflower seeds and almond slivers.

12. Make better choices at the salad bar by skipping the iceberg lettuce—it's almost entirely devoid of nutrition—and selecting the darker greens, such as romaine, red tip, Boston, Bibb and spinach. Top this off with vegetables that have dark yellow, orange and green colors, such as peppers, broccoli and squash. As a rule of thumb, the darker the color of the vegetable, the more nutrients it contains. Also, you can always:

• Sprinkle raisins on salads for fiber.

• Top any salad with shredded cabbage. It kicks in vitamin C and fiber.

• Get more copper by adding a few boiled shrimp, sesame seeds, nuts or mushrooms. Copper keeps bones, skin and tendons healthy and may reduce LDL cholesterol and boost HDL (high-density lipoprotein) cholesterol, the good kind.

• Avoid creamy dressings, most of which are loaded with fat. Instead go for vinegar or lemon with a little olive oil.

13. Power up tacos by increasing the carbohydrates and fiber. Swap canned pinto beans and brown rice for the beef. Here's our favorite recipe.

Coat a large skillet with cooking spray and heat. Sauté one small minced onion and two minced garlic cloves. Then add some chili powder, a pinch of cumin, ¼ cup of tomato sauce and ¾ cup of water. Bring to a boil, then add a can of drained pinto beans and a cup of quick-cooking brown rice. Cover and simmer for five minutes. Then remove from heat and let stand another five minutes. Spoon into taco shells or tortillas and top with low-fat grated Cheddar, hot sauce and shredded lettuce.

14. Popcorn is one of the healthiest snacks you can eat. A handful of air-popped popcorn has just six calories and is a good source of B vitamins and fiber. Make it even better by sprinkling on a tablespoon of brewer's yeast, available at health-food stores. Brewer's yeast adds B vitamins and a good dose of potassium. Also add garlic or chili powder for flavor.

15. Make a better burger by combining the beef one-to-one with mashed firm tofu in a mixing bowl. (You won't even taste the tofu, and you'll be adding B vitamins and calcium.) Next add chopped onion and whole-wheat bread crumbs for fiber. Mix in some egg white, a little ketchup and dried oregano. Form into patties and cook. Serve it on a whole-wheat roll and top it with romaine lettuce and tomato.

16. Want some fries to go with the burger? Try zucchini fries. Slice two zucchini into fry-size pieces. Sauté the fries in ½ teaspoon of oil in a large pan over medium-high heat until lightly browned. Sprinkle with basil. Or if you like things hot, sprinkle with Cajun spices.

17. Make a better barbecue with fish in place of meat. Not only is fish a good source of protein, it also contains omega-3 fatty acids, a good-for-you type of fat that may ward off heart disease. Fish also contains magnesium, B vitamins and potassium. Best fish for grilling: tuna, salmon, red snapper, halibut, bluefish and swordfish.

18. Grill leaner by cooking a turkey. Buy a thick, palm-size slab of turkey tenderloin, which is the leanest cut on the bird. Marinate it in a bowl of bottled low-fat Italian

salad dressing for ten minutes. Toss on the grill over high heat to brown both sides for about three minutes a side. Heat up an individual round pizza shell in a toaster oven for two minutes. Then wrap the shell around your turkey fillet, sandwichlike, and top with chunky salsa.

19. Get all the pleasure of apple pie with apple crisp instead. You gain cholesterol-lowering oats, and you lose almost all the fat. Here's an easy recipe.

Peel, core and slice eight medium-size apples and place them in a baking bowl coated with no-stick spray. In a separate bowl, mix together ½ cup of raisins, two tablespoons of lemon juice, ¾ cup of whole-wheat flour and 1¼ cups of oats. Drizzle with ½ cup of apple juice, ⅓ cup of honey or brown sugar and two tablespoons of canola oil, and add one teaspoon of cinnamon. Sprinkle this mixture over the apples and bake at 350° for about 30 to 40 minutes or until the apples are tender. Serve with a topping of vanilla frozen yogurt.

60-Second Power Boosters

Here are 11 more quick techniques for taking your meals to another level, nutritionwise.

20. Nearly double your intake of calcium and protein from a glass of milk, without adding fat. Mix two tablespoons of nonfat dry milk in an eight-ounce glass of cold skim milk. It'll make the skim milk thicker, too.

21. Power-pack prepared soups by adding a can of beans or crushed tomatoes to the simmering pot. Increase fiber by adding barley to vegetable soups.

22. Try fruit spreads on your toast instead of butter. Apple butter spread, for example, offers 38 milligrams of potassium per tablespoon and virtually no fat.

23. Substitute frozen melon balls for ice cubes in fruit drinks. One-half cup of honeydew melon has 230 mil-

ligrams of potassium and 20 milligrams of vitamin C.

24. Trim the fat off stews and soups by cooking them a day early and chilling them overnight. In the morning, skim off the fat.

25. Eat fruits and vegetables with their skins and peels intact for more fiber. For the same reason, eat the membranes that cling to oranges and grapefruit when you peel them.

26. Bread chicken breasts with bran cereal before baking them to load some fiber into the meal.

27. Add a handful of fresh parsley to stews, soups and sauces for a punch of beta-carotene.

28. Keep a bag of frozen corn in your freezer and use it to add fiber and carbohydrates to any meal. Toss ½ cup into whatever's cooking to add 17 grams of carbohydrates and 1.6 grams of dietary fiber.

29. Fling a handful of soy grits—available in health-food stores—into chili and stews. Soy adds B vitamins, calcium and zinc. And you'll hardly know it's there.

30. Raise calcium levels by sprinkling skim-milk powder into mashed potatoes, gravies and sauces.

—Margo Trott

All-Day Energy for On-the-Go Guys

Fight fatigue with this power-eating plan.

Your company certainly expects a lot for those jumbo bucks it pays you. Sixty-hour weeks, business trips on weekends, decision-intensive, nerve-splintering workdays. You need plenty of mental and physical stamina to get through it all. A proper diet can help. The problem is time. Who has enough to keep up with all the latest nutritional advice, gather the necessary ingredients of a healthy eating regimen and carefully ingest said ingredients at the right moment and in the correct amounts? When it comes to nutrition, what you want are the fast facts: What do I need to eat so that I can function at maximum efficiency? How can I eat it in a way that will waste the least amount of time?

To the busy man, the concept of three nutritious meals a day is little more than a fairy tale. Unpredictable working hours, surprise business lunches and deadlines that should have been met yesterday all conspire to keep you from maintaining anything close to the eating schedule your body and mind require to operate like a lean, mean living machine. But even if you do manage to get in those three squares, you could be falling short.

"One of the most important stamina rules is that your body needs its fuel in moderate doses throughout the day to keep energy nutrients optimally available at the cellular level," says Peter M. Miller, Ph.D., executive director of the Hilton Head Health Institute and author of *The Hilton Head Executive Stamina Program.* "I actually counsel people to eat between four and five times a day."

At first you might think that following this advice would make you a fat man rather than an energized one. But if we use an analogy Dr. Miller is fond of, the logic becomes a bit more apparent. Think about your car. Do you fill it up only after it runs out of gas? Or do you quite sensibly top off the tank at regular intervals, making sure that you always have enough fuel to go the distance?

"Many executives will grab a cup of coffee and a Danish around 8:00 A.M. and then put off lunch until 2:00 P.M. Meanwhile, they run out of gas by midday and spend a couple of hours operating at well below their peak stamina levels," notes Dr. Miller. "By eating four to five times a day, you avoid running low."

This isn't meant to give you a license to stuff yourself regularly. After all, you don't try to cram ten gallons of gas into your car when you need only five to fill the tank. "What I am suggesting is that you reduce the amount of food you eat at any one time so that you can spread the same amount of calories more evenly over the day," says Dr. Miller.

Eating less, but more frequently, makes good sense for another reason. "The larger the meal, the more time it takes to digest," says Dr. Miller. "And the process of digestion requires increased blood and oxygen flow to the stomach and intestines. This represents energy that will not be available for the brain and muscles to use." In other words, the bigger the meal, the more time you'll spend operating in that groggy, after-the-Thanksgiving-feast state of mind. It's not where you want to be when you have important decisions to make after lunch.

While your fueling schedule is an important component of your stamina level, the kind of fuel you use also makes a difference. A high-octane diet is one that is high in complex carbohydrates like those found in whole grains and vegetables.

"To ensure that you are receiving the large amounts of glucose that your body needs to maintain maximum energy, your basic fuel mix should be 60 percent carbohydrates, 15 percent protein and no more than 25 percent fat daily," says Dr. Miller. "Many people subscribe to the old belief that protein is where you get your energy, but this is not exactly true. Depend on foods such as vegetables, cereals, pastas, breads, potatoes and fruits to give you the carbohydrates your body needs to manufacture a steady supply of glucose. Rather than having a steak and fries for lunch, for example, you would do much better ordering a fruit platter, salad or perhaps pasta primavera. Fewer calories, more carbohydrates is the rule."

Late afternoon or midmorning (assuming you eat breakfast at 7:00 A.M. and lunch at 1:00 or 2:00 P.M.) is when you want to go for the additional mini-meal or snack. Dr. Miller suggests any of the following for a perfect pick-up when your glucose levels are sagging.

1 medium banana
1 orange
¼ cup raisins
5 dates
¼ honeydew melon
½ medium cantaloupe
3 medium apricots
½ medium apple
2 figs

To counteract dehydration, be sure to drink fluids throughout the day. "One of the things we know about energy is that when your body loses fluid, you tend to get tired," says Dr. Miller. "Executives should take particular care, since they frequently become dehydrated due to stuffy work environments as well as time spent in airplanes."

But you do want to go easy on coffee, colas and other caffeine-laden beverages. "Since caffeine is a diuretic, those drinks will only aggravate the problem." He suggests a "stamina spritzer": 60 percent orange juice and 40 percent carbonated water, served very cold. It also makes a good drink to help get you started in the morning, he says.

In the quest for stamina, many a man may wonder if some additional vitamins are in order. "My feeling," says Dr. Miller, "is that a well-rounded diet is the most important source of nutrients. But if you feel that you're guilty of some rather patchy eating habits, you may need to take a multivitamin with a mineral supplement for nutritional insurance."

In short, Dr. Miller's eating program for busy men is this: small, nutrition-packed meals, plenty of healthy snacks, a preponderance of complex carbohydrates, increased fluid intake and a multivitamin/mineral supplement if necessary.

—Mark Golin

All the President's Menus

Bill Clinton can tax himself all he wants, but he still can't balance his fat budget. Here's how you can balance yours.

In an ongoing effort to ensure domestic tranquillity, recent administrations have treated us to a stream of images designed to show off our presidents' virility. For four years, George Bush jogged, raced around in boats, played golf—anything to prove his fitness and lay aside fears that Dan Quayle might suddenly become president. Before that, Ronald Reagan chopped wood in his backyard, displaying his own vim and vigor and trying to quell fears that one day George Bush might become president.

The current talismans of presidential fitness are the constant photos of Bill Clinton running through the streets of Washington with a dozen panting G-men and a couple of visiting celebrities in tow. But the almost daily images of the 205-pound Clinton in his sweat-soaked jogging attire make one wonder—if this guy is so into exercise, how come he's still so heavy? Why do his joint press conferences with Boris Yeltsin look more like sumo wrestling matches than summit meetings? Why can't Bill Clinton lose that weight?

Slimming Down the Big Enchilada

To prove how pain-free fighting fat can be, we made a few tasteful substitutions in one of Bill Clinton's favorite dishes—chicken enchiladas. He likes them the way they're prepared at one of his Arkansas haunts, Trio's: filled with cheese and topped with a gooey cream sauce.

A traditional enchilada recipe calls for dipping the tortillas briefly into hot fat, then dipping them into the sauce and wrapping the chicken, onions and cheese with them. They are then placed in a well-oiled pan, covered with more sauce and baked for ten minutes. They're served topped with sour cream. Sounds delicious, until you look at the stats: Two enchiladas provide you with 925 calories, 57 percent of which come from fat, and 142 milligrams cholesterol.

Now take the simple substitutions we offer and try this: Warm the tortillas in an oven, without oil, and spray the baking pan with no-stick spray. For the sauce, sauté the onions and garlic in water or stock instead of oil. The results: 590 calories, 30 percent fat and 95 milligrams cholesterol.

There's a lesson to be learned here, and it's basically this: You can exercise until you wear holes in the soles of your cross-trainers, but unless you're smart about what you eat, you won't get that belly under control. And just because you're president, that doesn't mean you know any more about nutrition than the average school board electee. Clinton's diet is like most Americans': heavy on the meat and always followed by dessert. He also likes to nosh at midnight. One presidential late-night snack reportedly consisted of

Old recipe	New recipe
1 whole chicken breast, poached	Same
¾ pound Monterey Jack cheese	Kraft Monterey Jack Lite
1 onion, chopped	Same
8 flour tortillas	8 corn tortillas
2 tablespoons vegetable oil	No-stick pan spray
1 cup sour cream	1 cup fat-free sour cream

Tomatillo sauce	Our sauce
1 onion, minced	Same ingredients, but
2 cloves garlic, minced	substitute water or stock
2 tablespoons vegetable oil	for oil
1½ cups fresh tomatillos	
1 can chopped green chilies	
1 jalapeño, chopped	
½ teaspoon sugar	
Salt	

cocktail shrimp, pastries, mango sorbet and French bread dripping with olive oil.

Not so healthy, but wait—can't you just work out a little harder to burn off all those extra calories? Kind of like spending your way out of a recession? Not really. This is a supply-side issue. Let's say, for example, you run three miles at a clip of about eight minutes each—approximately President Clinton's pace on an average weekday. Then you stop at McDonald's and order up a Big Mac. What you've just done is burn off 384 calories, then immediately pile 500 back on.

Now, everybody knows that this is not good. In order to lose weight, you need to burn off more calories than you take in. So one might logically think "If I eat less food, I'll reduce the number of calories I'm taking in, and in no time I'll be fitting into those size 32 jeans I wore to peace marches at Oxford in 1968." Sorry, Bubba—not even if you inhale. In fact, strict diets are for chumps. The best way for any man to lose weight is to eat more, not less. As long as you eat more of the right things.

That's because your body is a highly evolved master-piece adept at keeping itself alive even during times of star-vation. And when you go on a diet, that's exactly what's happening—you're starving yourself. According to nutrition experts, diets don't work because when you deprive your body of food, your metabolic rate—the speed with which you burn calories—actually drops as the body tries to fight off what it thinks is starvation. So instead of using up your extra fat, your body clings to your love handles, unwilling to let them go lest the famine continue.

So the key is not to eat less but to eat less of the foods that make you fat and more of the foods that keep your metabolism revving. For example, let's say you and the president have diets that are about 40 percent fat—that's the average for Americans. Every gram of fat you eat comes jam-packed with nine weighty calories. By contrast, protein and carbohydrates have only four calories per gram. That means that for every gram of fat you cut out of your daily diet, you can add twice as many grams of carbohydrates and still be eating fewer calories. More food, fewer calories. Get it?

But replacing fat with carbohydrates works for another reason. Your body loves to convert dietary fat into body fat, because the transformation takes almost no energy. On the other hand, your body burns up almost ten times as many calories converting protein or carbohydrates into body fat. So it instead uses all the grains, fruits and vegetables for immediate energy and waits for that evening slice of cheesecake to make its way into your belly. A moment on the lips, a lifetime on the hips, as they say.

The question remains, how does one cut down on fat without destroying the pleasure of eating? We wouldn't put the commander in chief on a diet of grapefruit, tofu and water, and we wouldn't ask you to go on one, either. You don't need to deprive yourself to eat healthy, says Martin Yadrick, R.D., a nutritionist and spokesperson for the American Dietetic Association. For example, let's say you're a certain leader of a certain Free World with an overachieving wife and a bizarre genetic resistance to male pattern baldness. Or you're just some guy. Either way, here are the easy-to-follow rules.

1. Remember that many foods are naturally low in fat and jam-packed with the nutrients and fiber you need to keep you running. Not that you should stuff yourself, but within reason you can pretty much eat all you want of the following foods.

- Grains, like pastas, breads, rice, oats, barley and cereals, as long as they haven't been weighted down with fat and sugar (Sorry, beer doesn't count as a barley product.)
- Beans and legumes, such as kidney beans, peas, black beans, lentils, pinto beans and so on
- All fruits
- Vegetables like potatoes, carrots, asparagus, peppers, sweet potatoes and even that bane of the Bush kitchen, broccoli

2. Cows are fat factories, so be moderate in your consumption of whole-milk dairy products. Look for skim

milk and low-fat versions of yogurt, cheese and sour cream. If you're drinking whole milk now, make the switch to skim gradually, starting with 2 percent milk and working your way down over a month or so. By the time you're done, skim will be just as satisfying as whole milk used to be.

3. When it comes to meat, most of us eat too much. Hard-liners suggest you cut out meat altogether, but if you can't live without an occasional roast-beef sandwich, at least cut down on your consumption as much as possible. Six ounces a day is the most you want, says Yadrick, and even that is pushing it, so don't think that if you have rice and beans tonight you can have a huge porterhouse this weekend. A three-ounce serving of meat should be about the size of a deck of cards.

Of course, not all meat dishes are created equal. Here are some guidelines.

• A painless way to cut down on meat is to look for dishes where meat is an ingredient, not the centerpiece of the meal. Examples include stir-fries, chili, spaghetti with meat sauce or stews.

• Poultry is generally lower in fat than red meat, but you have to know your bird. Meat from the breast is less fatty than dark meat from the legs or wings, and removing the skin will cut a considerable amount of fat. Avoid fried chicken like the plague.

• When eating fish, steamed or broiled is your best bet. As for shellfish, choose those that don't swim, such as clams, mussels, scallops and oysters. They are the vegetarians of the sea, and as a result they are lower in fat than lobster, shrimp or crab.

4. Beware of oils of all kinds. That includes oil-containing products, such as margarine and most salad dressings. Remember that all oils are liquid fat—even olive oil,

safflower oil and canola oil. Look out for these hidden sources of oil: avocados, olives, nuts and seeds.

5. If you're taking the easy way out and buying prepackaged foods, look for low-fat products like Healthy Choice frozen meals, Health Valley chili (and many other Health Valley products), Kraft Free nonfat mayonnaise and salad dressings, Guiltless Gourmet tortilla chips, Quaker Oats oatmeal, Nabisco fat-free crackers, Fleischmann's Egg Beaters, Pritikin soups, Light n' Lively Free nonfat sour cream, Häagen-Dazs frozen yogurt bars and Entenmann's fat-free desserts.

Remember, your weight is primarily influenced by how much fat you eat, not how many miles you run. But with a few modest changes in your choice of fuel, you could be as fit and trim as Al Gore. So next time you jog all sweaty into a fast-food joint, remember this key phrase: "It's the fat, stupid."

—*Stephen Perrine*

Part Four

De-stress Your Tummy Away

Calm Down and Shed Pounds

Learning to bounce back from stress is a powerful way to shrink potbellies.

Those pounds of stress weighing on your shoulders . . . you feel them, even though you can't actually see them. But maybe you're looking in the wrong place. It could be they've migrated south—down to your potbelly.

This unexpected suggestion comes from researchers in the Department of Psychology at Yale University. And it could help explain why some people have more trouble with their midsections than they apparently deserve.

The Yale team believes that uncontrolled stress could be triggering the release of the hormone called cortisol, which in turn causes fat to be preferentially deposited around your middle.

Now, what exactly is "uncontrolled" stress? It's not the stress of doing a very challenging task and doing it well; rather, it's the stress of trying your best and failing repeatedly. It's not knowing what dreadful thing is going to happen to you next, or why. Most of all, it's a feeling that you just can't measure up, be in control, be on top. The kind of stress that's purely negative.

Researchers at Yale worked with 42 overweight women, ages 18 to 42. Some carried a preponderance of their overweight around their middles, others didn't. During tests, these women were given stressful tasks like being rushed through math problems and making speeches—during which they were falsely told their performances were poor. At the very same time, their levels of cortisol were measured. Women who carried their overweight in their bellies were secreting notably more of the stress hormone while under pressure. Readings taken the next day—with no special stressors—showed no unusual elevation of cortisol.

Backing up the connection, the women with the relatively larger bellies were also found to have less self-control.

In other words, it's not the stress itself but how you cope with it.

"This is the first time this chain of events has been shown in humans," researcher Marielle Rebuffe-Scrive, Ph.D., told us. She and colleague Judith Rodin, Ph.D., have been investigating this relationship between stress and abdominal fat for some time. Earlier work was largely based on animal experiments, one of which clearly demonstrated that lab rats subjected to stresses they can't control tend to get fat—especially in their tummies. So the new research findings are not exactly a surprise—the biological link between stress and the potbelly syndrome have already been made.

It's important to mention that fat carried on the belly, as opposed to the hips and thighs, has much more than aesthetic importance. As many *Prevention* magazine readers already know, the potbelly syndrome is strongly associated with an increased risk of heart disease, stroke and diabetes.

So banishing that pot—or preventing a future outcropping—is something that's surely worth doing even if your body's geography doesn't wound your self-image. It may mean living a longer, healthier life. The added benefit—fit-

Tune In to Breathing

Prevention magazine advisor Redford B. Williams, M.D., who is director of the Behavioral Medicine Research Center at Duke University Medical Center in Durham, North Carolina, suggests this simple routine to help get the *un-* out of uncontrolled stress. "There are some older studies from the early days of meditation research by a fellow named Ron Jevning, Ph.D., at California State University, Long Beach. His work showed that cortisol levels go down with transcendental meditation," says Dr. Williams.

Here are Dr. Williams's instructions for the everyday meditation. "Just pay attention to your breathing. Every time you breathe in and out, you notice it. Every time you breathe out, you say a word or phrase to yourself that conjures up the mental image you're trying to achieve, like 'Calm down, cool it,' for example. When your mind starts to wander and you're back thinking about whatever it is that was bugging you, just say to yourself 'Oh, well,' and come back to paying attention to your breathing and saying the word or phrase. To build your meditation skills, you need to practice for about ten minutes at least once a day. Then you will be able to meditate well and you will be able to call on these skills—when you're in a traffic jam, sitting there stewing, when you're angry at somebody or worried about something. This puts you in control."

ting into a slinkier negligee or a sleeker two-piece bathing suit—is just fat-free icing on a low-fat cake!

Now, you may be wondering if trying to get a better grip on your stress-control handlebars can actually help shrink your equators.

"Yes, we really suspect this might help," says Dr. Rebuffe-Scrive. "No, it's not going to be the single answer to make women lose all their abdominal fat. There are many causes of abdominal fat."

But, she adds, since high levels of poorly handled stress are also risk factors for several health problems—heart disease, for instance—it's definitely smart to try improving this area.

"Try to think," she says, " 'Why am I under stress? Why is this happening?' " Understanding the source of stress is the first step to dealing with it, "which everyone must find her own way to do," says Dr. Rebuffe-Scrive.

Our number one suggestion for combating stress is regular, enjoyable exercise. Exercise is often reported by individuals—like *Prevention* Walking Club members—to reduce stress and help you cope. Plus, walking—like any exercise—tends to burn belly flab for energy, so this is a two-way health and shape improver.

In addition to controlling stress, be sure to cut back on fat in your diet, exercise regularly and avoid serious drinking. You're bound to be healthier, and with any luck, you'll see your waistline shrink, too!

—Mark Bricklin with Michele Toth

Change Your Thinking and Shake the Weight

Here's how to weed out negative thoughts and cultivate a positive body image.

It's not life's hard knocks—in and of themselves—that make you sad or worried or angry. "It's more the way you interpret an event than the event itself that affects your mood. In all situations, it's what you're telling yourself that creates your emotions," says David D. Burns, M.D., clinical associate professor of psychiatry at the Presbyterian Medical Center of Philadelphia and author of *10 Days to Self-Esteem*. And that's very good news, he says, because we all have the ability to change how we look at the events in our lives.

It might help to think of your mind as a garden in which your thoughts can bloom. Some of those thoughts bring you delight and make you happy or confident. Others are like weeds. They strangle your happiness, making you feel inadequate or anxious. Your task is to yank the weeds and fertilize the thoughts that bring you self-confidence and joy.

Dr. Burns calls the weeds in your mental garden distorted or twisted thoughts. "Most of the thoughts that make you feel bad are distorted and unrealistic.

They're simply not true," he says. "They have been acquired over a lifetime and have become almost automatic. It will take some time and persistence to identify and change those thoughts. But it can be done, and it will change the way you feel!"

Here are strategies gleaned from psychologists, psychiatrists and educators to help you do this. Not all of the techniques described here will be equally helpful for you. As Dr. Burns says of his own techniques, "Different people, with different thoughts, find different techniques helpful." Among them all, you're likely to find advice that speaks to you.

But first a word of caution: These simple techniques for changing how you feel can be remarkably effective, even for serious depression. But you should definitely seek professional help, says Dr. Burns, if your negative feelings persist, if you've been unsuccessful in your efforts to overcome a mood problem and you feel stuck or if you have any suicidal or self-destructive thoughts.

Stop Those Twisted Thoughts

All of Dr. Burns's strategies for feeling better revolve around identifying and then changing distorted thoughts that make you upset. The four strategies that follow are designed to help you replace twisted thoughts with more realistic ones. "It takes practice to come up with realistic, convincing, valid and effective new thoughts that put the lie to your distorted ones," says Dr. Burns. "But don't think that it will be difficult or impossible for you."

Research by Dr. Burns and his colleague, clinical psychologist Jacqueline Persons, Ph.D., reported in the journal *Cognitive Therapy and Research,* found that it doesn't matter if you're rich or poor, brilliant or average, old or young, well-educated or not. Changing your thoughts has a huge impact on how you feel.

Examine the evidence. Let's say you're responsible for planning an event at your church, and it doesn't go well. Afterward, you tell yourself "I never do anything right. I'm such a loser." Now's the time to examine the evidence, says Dr. Burns. "Is it really true you never do anything right? Aren't there some things you actually do quite well? It may be that this event didn't go well, and you can learn from the experience. This makes you human, but certainly not a loser."

Do an experiment. "I was working with a lawyer who had this belief that if he ever lost a case, his colleagues would look down on him, and his career would vanish," says Dr. Burns. "He'd only ever lost a few cases. So I suggested that he do an experiment to test this belief. He agreed to describe one of the cases he'd lost to see what the reaction would really be at the next bar association meeting.

"He was amazed to discover his colleagues were not the least bit critical of him for his failure. In fact, they were grateful to learn he'd lost a case, and they opened up about their own problems. He felt closer to them than he ever had before. That's one of the great paradoxes: When you accept your shortcomings instead of hiding them in shame, they can become your greatest successes."

Think in shades of gray. Many of us think in absolute terms, says Dr. Burns—a total failure, or an absolute disaster. But in fact, there are always shades of gray. "Take my table-tennis game the other night. I don't win 100 percent of the time, but I don't lose 100 percent, either. Thinking in shades of gray, I can say I'm further along than I was three weeks ago, but I still have many skills to develop. It's a realistic way to look at things. Events are always a mixture of good and bad—never just one or the other."

Don't apply a double standard to yourself. Would you say the negative things you tell yourself to dear friends when they're feeling down? asks Dr. Burns. Of course not! "So talk to yourself the way you talk to others. I've found that most people who are depressed are a lot more reasonable and generous toward someone else than toward themselves."

Embrace Your Inner Critic

"There's a radio station playing in your head," say Hal Stone, Ph.D., and Sidra Stone, Ph.D., co-authors of *Embracing Your Inner Critic*. "We call it radio station K-R-A-Z-Y. It constantly broadcasts a running monologue of self-critical statements like 'That was a stupid thing to do,' or 'I'm so dumb,' or 'I'm not as good as they are.' Some people mistakenly think that inner critic is themselves. But it's not you. It's a voice inside of you that was preprogrammed at an early age to help you avoid rejection and shame by criticizing and correcting your behavior before other people could reject or criticize you first.

"You'll never eliminate or please your inner critic. But you can separate yourself from the self-criticism and keep it from dominating your thoughts and feelings," say the Stones. Here are their strategies.

Tune in to radio station K-R-A-Z-Y. Many of us aren't even consciously aware of that critical litany running in our heads. So the first step is to "pay attention to the things you say about yourself that you take for granted," say the Stones. "Catch yourself when you look disapprovingly at your face in the mirror. Take note when you start reviewing your day in the car on the way home from work, cataloging your mistakes and telling yourself how you could have done better." It may be easier if you record your inner critic's comments in a notebook.

Give your inner critic a face and name. Draw a picture of your inner critic, say the Stones, and give it a name. "This reinforces the idea that the inner critic is not you. It's a voice in your head. And it inserts a little needed humor and takes away the power of your inner critic to disturb or rule you." Dr. Hal Stone calls his inner critic Lothar the All-Powerful. Some people, he says, name their critics after critical people in their lives and give them recognizable faces. Others make them into dragons, demons or monsters.

Identify the voice of your inner critic. Who does your inner critic sound like? Does it sound like a parent, grandparent or teacher—or a combination of all of them? Trace it back to that person or persons who helped program your inner critic. This will demystify it even further, reducing its power over you.

Notice when your critic attacks come. Do your critic attacks come at regular times, maybe when you need to eat, or when you're tired, or when you're with someone you think is better than you in some way? Identify those people or moments that trigger your critic. It will help you manage your critic more effectively.

Stop the "incomparable comparer." "We're constantly faced with images in magazines and movies, and in the people around us, that tell us we ought to be fantastic and special. This makes our inner critic feel anxious, desperate and driven to be special or perfect—that 'incomparable comparer,' " say the Stones. "Remember that these destructive comparisons are being made by your inner critic, and you don't have to play the game."

Pull the Cork on Your Worries

"It's ironic," says Daniel Wegner, Ph.D., a professor of psychology at the University of Virginia in Charlottesville who specializes in overcoming unwanted thoughts and anxieties. "My research shows that the more you try to suppress unwanted thoughts, the more likely you are to become obsessed with them. That's particularly true when you're under a lot of pressure, stress or mental overload. So just when you're trying to avoid unhappy thoughts, you'll actually get sadder than if you confronted those unhappy thoughts head-on."

Dr. Wegner recommends the following strategies for keeping your worries in check.

Relax your control. Feeling depressed? "Give up trying to stop those unhappy thoughts," says Dr. Wegner. "The mental energy you're using to suppress them is keeping them just below the surface. When you lose control, the unwanted thoughts immediately surface, with even more power to distress you. But if you willingly relax control and let yourself think the thoughts you've been trying to avoid, it tends to relieve the pressure and power of those thoughts."

Schedule worry sessions. Dr. Wegner says research on chronic worriers has shown that if they spend an hour a night actively worrying about their problems, the degree of worrying in their lives goes down overall. "There's something boring, after all, about thoughts you spend an hour a night thinking about!" says Dr. Wegner.

Talk to a friend. "When you talk about your worries, it deflates those worries. They can't be suppressed. The cat's out of the bag, and thank goodness, it is just a cat, not some horrible monster," says Dr. Wegner.

Take Charge of Your Feelings

"Most people tell themselves 'I'm upset because that person cut in front of me in line' or 'because my husband doesn't understand.' Always because of something outside themselves," say Ron Hulnick, Ph.D., and Mary Hulnick, Ph.D., co-directors of the University of Santa Monica in California and members of the advisory board of the National Council on Self-Esteem. "But that idea doesn't work, because it means you always have to wait for an outside event to make you feel okay—and you may not have any control over those events." The Hulnicks recommend the following strategies to help you focus on what you can control—your reaction to those events.

Take 100 percent responsibility for what you're feeling. "When you blame someone else for how you're feeling," say the Hulnicks, "you give them the power to cause an emotional reaction inside of you. But when you take full responsibility for how you're feeling, the power comes back to you." Practice thinking this way, they say, and you'll start to realize that you have choices. You're not a victim of external circumstances.

Press the "cosmic delete button." We all have a strong tendency to judge ourselves, say the Hulnicks. "We tell ourselves we're incompetent because we didn't meet some level of expectation. We even judge ourselves for judging ourselves. But fortunately, we have a 'cosmic delete button' wired into our psychological system that can erase the judgment. It's called forgiveness.

"Here's how to use it: First, tell yourself that you want to be more aware of the judgments you make. Next, whenever you become aware that you've judged, forgive yourself. The more you do this, the more aware you become. It won't be too long before you begin catching yourself before you make judgments."

Write a letter. Here's an especially good technique to use when you're feeling angry: Just sit down with a pencil and paper and write a letter. "Maybe you're really angry about something a spouse or co-worker did. So write to them. Let it all out. Don't try to censor yourself. Don't worry about grammar, spelling or punctuation. Just keep writing what you're feeling. You'll know when you're done because you'll run out of steam.

"Next, burn the letter immediately, without rereading it. You've just had an emotional release, and rereading it only tends to inflame you all over again. You want to release the anger, not hang on to it."

Once you've let go of the anger, you'll be ready to deal constructively with the triggering situation.

Look for the lessons. There are two basic ways to look at a situation, say the Hulnicks: You can judge it and assign right or wrong to it. But judging usually makes you angry at others or upset with yourself. Or you can evaluate it—look at it objectively to see what you can learn from it.

"Everyone and every situation in life is a potential teacher. Situations you move through easily represent lessons already learned, while situations you react to with confusion, anger or fear are lessons still to learn.

"Looking at life this way isn't easy, but it is incredibly liberating and helps free you from the tendency to blame, shame or get one up on others. To start living life this way, all you need to do is ask yourself two questions for every situation: 'What can I learn from this?' and 'How can I improve what's going on here?' "

Who Are You Afraid of, Anyway?

Susan Jeffers, Ph.D., a psychologist and the author of many books and tapes, including *Feel the Fear and Do It Anyway* and *Dare to Connect*, likes to point out that 99 percent of what we worry about never happens. "So why not be realistic?" she says. "Feel the fear. That's part of being human. But go out and do things anyway, knowing that most of your fears are unfounded."

Dr. Jeffers says, "There's a chatterbox, a little voice inside our heads that's always heralding doom and disaster, breeding fear and uncertainty and defeat, even before we get started on something." But there are ways to keep that inner chatterbox from bringing you down, she says.

Outtalk your chatterbox. "Don't let that little voice take over," says Dr. Jeffers. "Consciously replace it with positive talk. Repetition is the key. You don't even need to believe what you're telling yourself, at first. Just talking positively changes our energy and helps us move forward."

One great tool in this effort, says Dr. Jeffers, is the use of affirmations—simple, positive statements repeated frequently: "There is nothing to fear." "I'm in control of my life." "Whatever life hands me, I'll handle it." "I let go and I trust."

Chart your path from pain to power. Your chatterbox creates pain, leaving you feeling helpless, depressed, frightened or paralyzed, says Dr. Jeffers. You really want just the opposite: to feel like you have choices, to feel excited about life and to feel capable of getting things done. As a visual reminder of this path you want to take, she suggests putting a skinny horizontal chart on your refrigerator. On the far left, put the word "pain," and on the far right, put the word "power." Connect the two words with a line. Next, put a movable magnet on the line to represent where you are now on the continuum. Each day, look at the chart and ask yourself if you see yourself in the same place or if you think you've moved.

"Awareness is half the battle," says Dr. Jeffers. "Before you take any action, ask yourself 'Is this action moving me to a more powerful and loving place?' The chart will motivate you to keep moving in the right direction, especially if you look at it as a fun process of growth and discovery."

Watch your words. "On the path from pain to power," says Dr. Jeffers, "it's important that you monitor your words, using phrases that empower rather than weaken you. So eliminate the can'ts, shoulds, problems and struggles from your vocabulary. Replace them with power words."

Expand your comfort zone. "Much of the time, we're afraid to move out of that zone of comfort we've decided is safe for us," says Dr. Jeffers. To break through the fears that limit us, take a small risk each day. Call someone you've

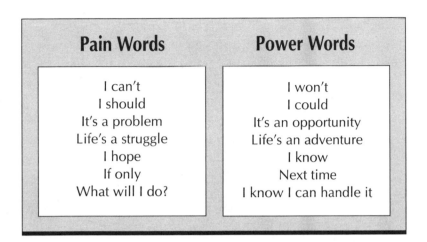

Pain Words	Power Words
I can't	I won't
I should	I could
It's a problem	It's an opportunity
Life's a struggle	Life's an adventure
I hope	I know
If only	Next time
What will I do?	I know I can handle it

been intimidated to call before. Ask for something you have always wanted but were afraid to ask for. "Even if it doesn't quite work out as you expected it to, at least you tried. You didn't sit back, powerless. And you will feel your confidence grow."

Consider the alternatives. "Each time you get upset or are confronted with a difficult situation, consider your alternatives," says Dr. Jeffers. Write down in a notebook all the possible ways you could act and feel—angry, happy, foolish, challenged, excited. "This demonstrates that you have the power to change your viewpoint, and your feelings, whenever you want to," says Dr. Jeffers.

Focus on others, not yourself. "Imagine you're standing in the doorway leading to a roomful of interesting strangers," Dr. Jeffers says. "In that situation, most of us are focusing on ourselves, on our fear of rejection or our fear of appearing foolish. But what if you turned the focus around and asked yourself 'How can I make someone in there feel good about themselves tonight?' understanding that everyone feels uncomfortable facing a roomful of strangers. That takes the fear out of a roomful of strangers. You'd become a 'giver,' not a 'getter,' leaving you in a more confident, less needy position. And if you do get rejected, your new feeling of confidence will assure you that you'll handle it, and you'll move on to someone else who would welcome your warmth and love."

Ride the Upward Spiral to Smarter Living

"Getting rid of a bad mood is not a trivial matter," says Adam Khan, a Washington-based writer and educator who conducts workshops and produces audiotapes on effective thinking and communication skills. "Improving your mood won't solve the serious or heartbreaking problems in your life. But when you elevate your mood, you make better decisions, which makes you feel better still, which makes you act more intelligently—which can set you on an upward spiral."

Here are some of Khan's favorite mood-boosting strategies.

Act as if . . . "Sometimes you want to act or feel differently, but you don't know how to do it. You feel stuck," says Khan. "So act as if you felt the way you want to feel. Assume the posture you would have if you felt the way you want to feel. Breathe the way you would breathe. Talk the way you would talk. Think the way you would think. Look the way you would look. When you act as though you're confident or cheerful, you begin to feel confident or cheerful. And after a while, it's no longer an act."

Clean up your integrity. "It's impossible to feel good about yourself when you think you've done something wrong," says Khan. "So the way to like yourself better is to clean up your integrity." Here's how to do that. First, make a list of what you're doing that you think is wrong, and simply stop doing those things. "Just making the list will give you some relief, because we're never as bad as we think we are." Next, make amends for things you've done in the past

Dieters Help Feed the Hungry

One candy bar per week seems like it's only a tiny expense—but over time that money spent amounts to enough rice, milk and peanut butter to feed a small family for a few months.

That's why a new program called Dieters Feed the Hungry is helping people channel their fatty expenses into the hungry mouths of the poor.

"We founded this to resolve a glaring paradox—that millions of people are dieting while many others don't have enough food to make it through the month," says Ronna Kabatznick, Ph.D., founder of the group in Oakland, California. "We encourage dieters to refocus their time and energy and money to worthwhile causes." The program gets scale watchers to donate food or volunteer time to a local agency and hooks them up with the neighborhood food bank or Red Cross.

"Helping others who are in need gives dieters an outlet for feelings of emptiness that may drive them to overeat," says Dr. Kabatznick. It's nice to lend a hand during the holiday season, too—but also offer your help at other times of the year when volunteerism isn't so popular.

For more information, you can write to: Dieters Feed the Hungry, P.O. Box 5604, Berkeley, CA 94705. Please include a self-addressed, stamped business-size envelope.

that you feel guilty about. It may need only an apology, or it may require an action that makes up for the damage. "This is never as bad as you think," says Khan. "In fact, it can really lighten your load and make it more fun to be alive." Finally, forgive yourself for all the bad things you've done.

Find the temporary cause. "When a setback or failure

Can Weight Be Talked Away?

Somewhere between the basement and the attic, you already have the device that may prevent your plump pre-teen from becoming an obese adolescent. It's called the rest of the family.

Most overweight kids balloon into their teens. But a new Swedish study showed that when parents and siblings got involved, overweight kids didn't gain as much weight. Researchers uncovered this when they gave 19 obese ten-year-olds exercise instructions and a low-calorie diet strategy. A group of 20 others got that strategy plus six sessions (over 18 months) of family therapy—talk sessions with the whole family and a family therapist that help everyone sort out what's working (or not working) in how the family functions. For instance, family members might learn how to problem-solve, nurture, set limits with one another and talk about feelings. By getting the family to work better together, the child receives not only the nurturing needed to prevent emotional overeating but also the limits required to develop a healthy lifestyle.

By the time the obese kids reached age 14, those whose clans helped out stopped the bulge, while everyone else gained weight. Based on this study, if an average, overweight 10-year-old (starting at 100 pounds) had family therapy in

really upsets and depresses you, it's probably because you think the cause of the failure is permanent. You think you can't change it no matter how hard you try," says Khan.

But what if you focused, instead, on the temporary, changeable causes? Maybe you were tired this week because of out-of-town visitors. That's a temporary problem. Or maybe you were overextended and really didn't have conjunction with behavioral treatment, he might reach his teens weighing 138 pounds. On diet and exercise alone, he might be closer to 145, but without anything, his weight could inflate to 150.

American researchers say this study is the first published evidence to confirm what they've suspected all along. "We've seen for some time that it's only when you have an impact on the family functioning that weight loss persists in the child for the long term," says Laurel Mellin, R.D., director of the Center for Child and Adolescent Obesity at the University of California, San Francisco. That's because family therapy doesn't just treat the pounds once they're on, she says. It also helps pull the plug on what's luring the child's hand to the cookie jar in the first place. That's why many child-obesity programs conducted by hospitals already weave together lifestyle and family therapy in caring for obese children.

The bonus for the household with a chunky child is that most families end up with more than a slim teen, says Mellin. "The whole family gets an opportunity to become closer. And parents find they feel better about their parenting." Check with your family doctor for information on how to find a program with a family therapist in your area.

the time. You can change that, too, by dropping activities or managing your time better. "Looking for the temporary causes to setbacks forms a new habit of thinking that lets you bounce back from adversities that would have laid you out flat before."

Ask yourself for advice. Feeling upset about something? Sit down and have a conversation with yourself on paper, says Khan. "Start by writing out your problem clearly. Then write a question, as if you were asking the wisest person in the world. Finally, answer your question on paper to the best of your ability. Imagine that your best friend was asking you that question and really wanted your answer. I think you'll be absolutely floored by how wise you are. You'll come up with brilliant solutions and feel better, too."

—Chris Hill with Toby Hanlon

Take the "Nature Cure" and Revitalize

How a walk in the woods provides the perfect antidote to midlife stress.

Remember, as a child, your secret garden or woodland cove—your private nature retreat? There, you could tell a tree or a star your innermost feelings without fear of judgment or rejection. You could go to this place and be yourself and feel accepted.

In the journey toward becoming grown up, many of us abandoned the wisdom of our youth. It wasn't intentional. We just got busy establishing and juggling careers, families and homes. By the time we got a free moment to look up from our "to do" lists, two, or even three, decades had whizzed by.

All too often, we arrive at midlife overworked and overwhelmed, with spirits that ache for more.

"In midlife, we become aware of the need for simplicity, the need to decompress," says Ross Goldstein, Ph.D., a San Francisco psychologist and recognized expert in the psychology of midlife and author of *Fortysomething*. "We desperately long to slow down the manic pace, tune out the clamor of demands and find a source of silence, tranquillity and rejuvenation."

119

How to Get a Spirit Lift from Nature

Between concrete walls, shopping malls and city halls, it's darn hard to find open space anymore. Top that with a hectic lifestyle, and no wonder communing with nature gets the squeeze. Luckily, there are creative ways to bring nature to your doorstep, even if you live in the city.

Take your fitness walks in a tranquillity zone. Instead of beating your feet along city sidewalks or suburban sprawls, treat yourself to a gentle path in a nearby woods or park. Tune in to the seasonal changes, the play of sunlight and shadows and the movement of wildlife.

Be a nature observer and explorer. Take a field guide with you on your wilderness walks and learn the indigenous birds and trees by name. Or discover a microworld of activity with a magnifying glass. Let the lens of a camera reveal new ways to look at familiar surroundings.

Get a dog. Rain or shine, Rufus gets you out of your four walls and into the open air. One inhabitant of Pasadena,

If only we would remember to turn our gaze to the awe of a child, we would recall that such a place exists within our grasp—in a garden, in a woods, by a stream. In nature, we would find what we're longing for: a beauty and stillness that let the extraneous fall away and allow the essence of who we really are to emerge.

Waking Up to Midlife

Like a tree sending roots deep into the soil, reconnecting with our true selves provides us with stability and equanimity in the face of midlife gusts.

California, swears, "I've never been more in touch with nature than since I got my dog."

Find a secluded spot, and sit and watch. At first, against the chaos of your mind's activity, it will seem that nothing is happening. But give the mental chatter time to wind down and your senses a chance to open up. Listen. Smell. Watch. Feel. Soon you'll begin to notice a fascinating universe of life around you.

Garden. Having even a small plot where you can dig, plant seeds and watch things grow is a powerful way of getting in synchronization with natural cycles. Window gardens can delight city dwellers, too.

Seek outdoor adventures close to home. Revive your thrill-seeking urge! Get the pink back in your cheeks with a refreshing challenge like tubing down a river or hitting local trails on a mountain bike. Cap off your invigorating day with a relaxing picnic.

"The three big wake-up calls of midlife are disconcerting," says Dr. Goldstein. "They include the realizations that, one, you're not going to become president of the company (or, if you are president, it's not as fun as you thought it would be); two, your family life is never going to look like Ozzie and Harriet's; and three, you're not going to live forever."

The good news is that these painful realizations can prompt positive change and propel us to a new level of personal growth and fulfillment.

"Everybody does some soul-searching in midlife, but the degree to which people reorganize their lives and make significant changes varies," says Dr. Goldstein.

"Typically, people ask themselves 'Where am I going with my life? What should I do?' But midlife isn't just about what you do; it's primarily about who you are," Dr. Goldstein points out. "If we wish to embrace the second half of life with renewed vitality and vigor, we must devote some quality time at midlife to reassessing who we've come to be and who we'd still like to become.

"That process, we know from experience, does not happen spontaneously," he explains. "The inner voice that holds the answers cannot be heard against the din of everyday static. In order to hear it, we must stop and intentionally carve out a little quiet, contemplative time."

Nature Readings

On those days when you can't get your RDA of nature in the great outdoors, these books can at least transport you in spirit.

Walden, **by Henry David Thoreau.** This personal account of the simple life on Walden Pond belongs on every nature-seeker's shelf.

Earth Prayers from around the World, **edited by Elizabeth Roberts and Elias Amidon.** A handy volume of prayers, poems and invocations honoring the earth.

The Sacred Landscape, **by Frederic Lehrman.** A beautiful, oversize photographic essay accompanied by inspiring poems.

Gift from the Sea, **by Anne Morrow Lindbergh.** In the story of her month at the seashore, Lindbergh exquisitely reveals how nature provides a model for intimate relationships.

Support from Mother Earth

Nature provides the perfect antidote to our hectic and complex existence.

"In the material, conventional world, we are pitting our own lives against a pace of existence that almost doesn't have room for our pace," says Mel Bucholtz, a therapist and co-director of the Returning to Earth Institute, which hosts wilderness trips. "When we go back to the natural world, we start to see a time sequence that we fit into. Instead of pressure, we feel acceptance." For once, we feel content not doing anything, just being.

"In the quiet of nature, you get the solitude and presence of mind to deal with the significant issues of your life," says Valerie Andrews, author of *A Passion for This Earth*. "It is when you allow the tide of your own activity to go out. And in the absence of all those activities, you gain wisdom and insight."

Compost for Personal Growth

Not only does nature free us from noise and distractions, the natural processes and rhythms also provide valuable insights into our personal transitions.

One of the most difficult tasks of the midlife transition is learning to let go of old, outmoded life structures in order to move on to new ones.

"When you talk to people who are beginning the process, they talk about loss, about the things they have to give up, not about what they're going to gain," says Dr. Goldstein.

"Saying good-bye to an unrealistic image of yourself, to your dreams that haven't panned out, to careers, to people—friends, spouses, parents—inherently carries pain," he

(continued on page 130)

Real-Life Lessons from Nature

Anne Grosser, 50

While I maintained an active career, my kids always came first. Then last year, my youngest daughter left for college. I was faced with the challenge of redirecting my energies from parenting her to "parenting" myself. Wanting to experience new adventures as my daughter was about to, I decided to do something just for me. I was nearing my 50th birthday, and I'd feared that turning 50 meant going around that bend to old age.

Determined not to surrender to my fears, I decided to do something special just for me, something I had never done and actually wouldn't even have considered doing before. I signed up for a ten-day backpacking/camping trip in New Mexico.

At this moment in my life, the idea of hiking in the wilderness seemed incredibly appealing. Living surrounded by concrete in New York City, my body yearned for pure air, open space and beautiful, natural surroundings. For me, too, a big part of the attraction was the physical challenge. Although I've never been athletic, I longed to feel that I was vital and strong.

In fact, nature proved to be more of a challenge than I imagined. The first day out, we backpacked to a base camp. It really wasn't that far in terms of miles—maybe a mile and a half. But we were climbing in a deep, evergreen forest, not the flat New Mexico desert terrain I had anticipated. And I had never carried so much! My backpack weighed 40 pounds. Despite practicing yoga and doing some weight lifting, I wasn't prepared for this. I burst into tears. I'd never felt so vulnerable in my life.

On day two, the earth offered more challenges. We hiked six or seven miles up the mountain. It was quiet, dotted with beautiful wildflowers, but the climbing was intense.

Breathing heavily, I sucked in the scent of pine.

As the oldest and slowest member of our group, I tended to fall to the back of the pack. At first, I tried to follow step-by-step in the footprints left in the soft, brown dirt by another hiker. I thought this would help give me a better grip. In fact, it threw me off balance because her stride was so different from mine. It occurred to me that this experience had a parallel in my life's journey; so often did I try to follow someone else's path, thinking it would be easier than carving my own way. I suddenly realized that in nature, as in life, I must create my own path.

As the trail became steeper and increasingly difficult for me to climb, my confidence faltered. I had to stop; for a moment, I didn't believe I could make it to the top with the others.

That's when Nancy Goddard, who led our group, offered me some words of encouragement. "The process of getting up the mountain is more important than the end result," she told me. "Just take it one step at a time."

To help me, she taught me the "grandmother step." That's where you take a teeny step, stop and take a deep breath, then exhale. Then you move the second foot and take a breath in and out, and so on. It's very slow, but it keeps you moving.

That, too, became a powerful metaphor in my own life. Instead of feeling overwhelmed by difficult challenges, I learned that by focusing on the process and tackling problems one teeny step at a time, the seemingly impossible is possible. I know that because the grandmother step enabled me to make it to the top of that mountain. And what an incredibly empowering experience that was!

Amazingly, every day offered me more insights. Our hiking journey took us across 17 streams. I was pretty appre-

(continued)

Real-Life Lessons from Nature—Continued

hensive about wading through the frigid water. At first, the iciness seemed unbearable. But as I released my discontent and simply accepted that this was part of the deal, I grew to relish the invigorating, tingling sensation in my legs. There was a freedom in letting go of my fears and negative expectations and allowing myself to just experience the moment.

No doubt about it: Toughing out those ten days in nature strengthened my body. And most important, in the process, I learned a lot about myself.

Dulanie Ellis-La Barre, 44

I grew up in Hollywood, a real city girl. In my thirties, I worked on my own as a corporate travel consultant, so I spent a lot of time on the phone. Then, after three years of trying to keep my business afloat during a recession, it was time for a change.

Financially and emotionally drained, I packed up my two cats and my dog and moved to a little seaside town north of Los Angeles. There my cousin had an old family beach house—a little ramshackle, one-bedroom clapboard place, right on the water. At her suggestion, I became a recluse there for a couple of months.

It was a blissful setting. No billboards. No neon signs. And, I couldn't believe my ears, the hum was gone. In the city, the silence is filled with an ever-present electrical hum. Amazingly, when I lived there, I never even noticed it.

At the beach, I discovered tranquillity. The rhythm of the ocean slowed me down. When I'd wake in the morning, the waves would be slapping at the seawall. By afternoon, the tide would be way out, and I could go tide-pooling for starfish.

Soon, I met a new friend, Douglas. Together we sailed to

the pristine Channel Islands just off the coast. We went exploring in sea caves, our dinghy escorted by dolphins. We saw sea lions and whales out in the channel. It was absolutely thrilling!

I've always been a very fearful person, terrified to try new things. The first time Doug took me snorkeling, I was paralyzed with fear. Just as I started to relax, I noticed what I thought was an anchor on the seafloor. In fact, it was a huge stingray! My fear propelled me out of the water and into the dinghy in one move!

Somehow, though, I had the courage to get back in the water. Afterward, I felt so empowered personally for having done that. Nature helped coax me out of my shell, extending my comfort zones, gently helping me believe more in myself.

One day, while hiking alone in the nearby hills, I came across a wonderful little creek, flowing around little islands of moss and water flowers. It was such an enchanting setting, I decided to sit a spell right in the middle of the stream on a rock.

As I sat quietly, watching the sun glimmer off the water, something totally unexpected happened: I began to sing. I started out a little subdued, but pretty soon I was belting it out, making up verse after verse. I must have gone on singing for an hour! Now, that may not sound like much, but if you knew me . . . I'm one of those people who doesn't sing, not even "Happy Birthday."

That event challenged my self-image in a very positive way. I realized that all those assumptions I held about myself—what I could and couldn't do—were no longer valid. As a result, I began to trust more in myself and in my relationships, especially with Douglas. When I was 41, we got

(continued)

Real-Life Lessons from Nature—Continued

married. And at 43, for the first time in my life, I felt secure and happy enough in who I am to have a child—a little girl.

Boni Hamilton, 41

Three years ago, when I began walking at dawn, I didn't expect to like any part of it. But desperate to lose the excess weight childbearing and age had added, I chose walking as an inexpensive exercise program. Besides, the early hour ensured me a free baby-sitter: my sleeping husband.

For the first month, I trudged four miles along suburban streets and counted the minutes until I could return home. The monotony of the tract houses, the unending chorus of barking dogs and the steady stream of cars left me tense and irritable. Exercising became a chore, and I resented it. Then my husband, John, suggested I walk on the Highline Canal, a 72-mile earthen irrigation ditch that meanders through the Denver metro area, in the shadow of the Rockies.

"At least there won't be any cars," he said, "and you can use the mileage markers to track your distance."

At first I enjoyed the change of scenery. I liked the variety of homes backed up to the canal. After a while, though, even these became familiar, and the novelty palled.

Walking is boring, I decided.

Then I discovered a new world: birds.

Magpies had always fascinated me. Their harlequin plumage made them easy to spot, and I loved to watch their feathers fan and slide as the birds rode air currents or landed in trees.

I hadn't paid attention to any of the other species that flitted among the trees, though. Now I noted specific characteristics of the birds I saw—color, body size, wing shape, song and habits. At home later, I consulted field guides and "birder" friends to identify what I had seen.

I watched the great blue heron fishing in the canal. Red-tailed hawks circled the meadow. Once I glimpsed a kestrel tucked in a willow only an arm's length from me.

This study of birds did not slow me down. I learned to sweep large areas in a glance and to notice even the tiniest movement. Walking became a challenge to find new curiosities.

One morning, I spotted three mule deer gliding single file toward a stream. I trailed after them until they disappeared among some trees. By then, I had gone a mile beyond my turnaround point and had no choice but to walk the extra distance back.

Surprisingly, walking those six miles seemed no more tiring than four. So I decided to go six miles every day.

Within two weeks, I knew my decision had been wise. I felt more energetic, and my rate of weight loss doubled. Best of all, the extra distance was even richer in wildlife.

In the spring when the canal was full of water, I stopped to investigate a soft splash and looked down on a beaver pulling grass from the bank. Foxes, both black and red, had dens along the canal. Often I'd catch glimpses of the white-tipped tail as a fox dived into brush, or I'd smell the distinctive musk, a fragmentary odor similar to a skunk's, that meant a fox had been there. Once I spotted a fox sitting by a lawn chair at the edge of a tennis court and looking, for a moment, like a family pet.

My favorite encounters, though, have been with coyotes. Unlike foxes, coyotes seem unafraid of people. On one occasion a coyote walked a quarter of a mile with me; only a grassy bank and a fence separated us.

I enjoy these encounters with nature so much that even though I lost the desired 30 pounds in five months, I have continued my regimen. My daily excursions do more than condition my body; they rejuvenate my soul.

continues. "But you have to say good-bye before you can say hello to whatever will be the next life structure that you're looking at."

"If you can't let go of those things and go into another cycle of risk and challenge, you just repeat the same thing over and over again and get stuck in old patterns of being," Andrews adds.

Nature helps people realize how to accomplish the transition. "Sitting next to a rotting stump, a person may notice new shoots growing out of the decay. That's a graphic example of transition," explains Bucholtz. "What people discover is that as things decay, compost is created to foster new growth."

Taking lessons from nature helps us more gracefully surrender to the natural ebb and flow of life.

"The process of moving around obstacles is reflected beautifully against the backdrop of a natural phenomenon like a river or a storm," Bucholtz says. "When you see how a river changes course to continue its flow, or witness the way a landscape recovers after a devastating storm, you see how you can work in the way nature does with regard to change."

Submitting to the natural order induces a tremendous sense of relief because we no longer have to fight it. We can simply go with the flow.

One with Nature

There's also something very comforting in knowing you're connected to the whole of nature. You're not outside of it; you're a part of it.

"In a way, a lot of people feel as though they're coming home when they're in the natural world," Bucholtz explains. "They belong in nature. They fit. They're an integral part of a system. That gives people we've seen a tremendous sense of personal relief."

"When I was going through my own midlife conflicts, I often rode my bike out to the ocean," says Dr. Goldstein. "I would be preoccupied trying to make decisions about my future, and I would look out at the ocean and say 'This has been here forever, and it's going to be here forever,' and soon the insignificance of my decisions would pale by comparison.

"At first, I'd feel my insignificance down in my gut. But then, that would be replaced by a tremendous comfort, a feeling of safety in just being a small cog in the larger works."

Awakening the Senses

Spending time in nature can also reinvigorate us by re-awakening our senses and our creative spirits.

"In the urban environment, people tend to be mostly in their heads. They don't use their senses and end up missing very important information," says Jackie Farley, president of CenterPoint, an Aspen, Colorado, retreat center for women. "In nature, we become more present, more mindful, more aware of our surroundings."

To bring that concept to life, participants in Farley's retreats hike the Braille Trail, a nature trail near Independence Pass designed for the blind. The group walks the trail twice, first blindfolded and then with eyes open.

"What we discover is that as we overuse one sense, such as our eyes, we shortchange information coming from the other senses," says Farley. "When blindfolded, we hear more, we feel the sun as we move in and out of it, we smell the rich earth. As we gain access to all our senses, we become whole again.

"I don't see how we can be fully aware of our power to make decisions and to listen to our intuition unless we learn to use all the parts of ourselves as sources of information."

"As the aesthetic senses reawaken, people begin to talk

about the reawakening of their sense of life in an almost artistic way," says Bucholtz.

Whether it's to invent an object, a painting, music, a social program, a new way of being in a relationship, whatever, people often feel inspired by the richness and diversity of the natural environment.

Regaining the creative impulse is a found treasure—something many claim they'd lost years ago.

The Physical Challenge

Inspiration can come from watching a sunset, a snowfall, a tree turned gold in autumn. But it can also come climbing a mountain or swimming against a swift river current. Meeting the physical challenges of nature has special meaning in midlife.

"We don't test our bodies very often," says Nancy Goddard, a leader of backpacking journeys into wilderness areas of the country. "A lot of people at midlife have given up on their bodies and succumb to aging without challenging themselves in a way that shows their physical strength and vitality."

As people then confront and triumph over physical challenges, they feel incredibly empowered emotionally as well, she adds. "Suddenly, they have a faith in themselves they didn't have before."

Dr. Goldstein agrees. "Tenacity as a character trait is ambiguous. But tenacity, as characterized by the ability to continue rowing a boat or hiking up a steep trail long past the point where you want to quit, is concrete. Seeing yourself in that light is very valuable." With nature to nurture us, midlife becomes a season of wonder and rejuvenation, when our lives really bear fruit.

—Sharon Stocker

Part Five
Cope with Cravings

Mastering the Monster

Ten guaranteed ways to curb the colossal cravings that can threaten even your best weight-loss efforts.

Like Godzilla, Frankenstein and the particularly loathsome Swamp Thing, cravings are a monstrous lot. They're gargantuan . . . slippery . . . even nefarious, and mere mortals usually fare poorly when faced with their evil doings. But as B-movie buffs will attest, celluloid monsters are not invincible—and neither are cravings. The key to success against the latter lies in following scientifically proven advice.

Researchers who study cravings have devised a relatively simple and effective plan of attack for dieters who want to hush their hankerings. What follows are ten scientifically proven ways to curb the urge to eat when it rears its monstrous head. Read on, and prepare for battle.

1. Drown your appetite. "Drinking generous amounts of water is the number one way to reduce your appetite," says George L. Blackburn, M.D., chief of the Nutrition/Metabolism Laboratory at New England Deaconess Hospital in Boston. Because oceans of water take up seas of space in your stomach, you'll feel full, which will quell the urge to eat. Aim to take in 64 ounces of fluids a day, sipping on 3- or 4-ounce glasses at a time.

2. Graze selectively. Most moms wouldn't recommend snacking before mealtime, but many scientists now do. For instance, James Kenney, R.D., Ph.D., a nutrition-research specialist at the Pritikin Longevity Center in Santa Monica, California, believes that nibbling small amounts of food throughout the day suppresses the appetite more than eating a few larger meals. Grazing, he says, keeps insulin levels steadier—and lower—than gorging. (High insulin levels stimulate the appetite and prompt fat cells to take in fat molecules instead of allowing your muscles to use them as energy.)

But to graze effectively, Dr. Kenney warns, you must munch the right kinds of foods. "You can't nibble on M & M's, potato chips and Häagen-Dazs," he says. "If you do, your insulin levels and appetite will increase. Grazing on low-fat, high-fiber foods that aren't packed with calories— such as carrots, peaches, oranges, red peppers, pastas, potatoes and oatmeal—will keep your appetite down." Eat healthful snacks, such as a bagel, a few raw baby carrots and a piece of fruit, once every two hours or so during the day.

3. Soup it up. Researchers at Johns Hopkins University in Baltimore compared soup with other appetizers to see which food did the best job of arresting the appetite. For two weeks, 12 men ate one of three first courses—tomato soup, Muenster cheese on crackers or fresh fruit—before a large lunch. Although each dish contained the same number of calories, tomato soup proved to be the most satisfying; the men tended to eat fewer calories at lunch after sipping soup than they did after munching on fruit or cheese and crackers.

Why is soup so satiating? Researchers speculate that it's

the large volume of space soup takes up in the stomach. (They ruled out warmth and salt content when they found that cold, low-sodium soup reduced appetite, too.) The fact that soup is high in carbohydrates, which release a brain chemical called serotonin that contributes to a feeling of well-being, may also contribute to soup's ability to satisfy.

Sip soup before large dinners or as a meal in and of itself. And opt for a tomato-based soup when you eat out—it's less fattening than mayo-laden salads or cream-based soups, and it'll fill you up better.

4. Load up on complex carbohydrates. Low-fat, high-carbohydrate foods, such as rice, potatoes and pastas, satisfy the appetite with fewer calories than high-fat foods, primarily because carbohydrates are easily converted to glycogen, whereas fat is not. And stored glycogen, which is the body's most important energy source, suppresses hunger. Compare, for instance, an ounce of potato chips with a baked potato. Each packs 160 calories, but the chips, which are laden with fat, are far less likely to fill you up than the baked spud, which is mostly carbohydrates.

What's more, if the carbohydrates you eat are derived from whole grains, fruits, vegetables and beans instead of processed sugars and starches, they will replenish glycogen stores without boosting insulin levels, which stimulate the appetite—and fat storage.

Carbohydrates are also digested and stored less efficiently than fat. "This means that your metabolic rate increases more when your body is processing carbohydrates than when it is metabolizing fat," says Dr. Kenney. "A higher metabolic rate produces more body heat, which is associated with a reduced appetite."

Another theory as to why carbohydrates dim the desire to eat involves serotonin. Because a lack of this brain chemical is linked with depression and because many people with the blues are also overweight, some scientists postulate that a lack of serotonin stimulates food cravings and that a surplus reduces hunger.

Whatever the reason for carbohydrates' satisfying effect, it works. Nutritionists recommend eating 6 to 11 daily servings of grains, such as breads, cereals and pastas. And because it can take up to 20 minutes for your appetite to slow after eating carbohydrates, try munching on a high-carb snack about 20 minutes before you sit down to a meal. Try whole-wheat bread (without butter), soup with noodles or rice or a small serving of spaghetti, and you'll probably wind up eating less food than you normally would in the long run.

5. Say *si* to spicy foods. Mexican, Thai, Szechuan and Indian fare fill you up more quickly than blander foods. "The flavor is so intense, you simply don't need as much to sate your appetite," explains Maria Simonson, Sc.D., Ph.D., director of the Health, Weight and Stress Clinic at Johns Hopkins Medical Institutions.

In addition, spicy foods speed up your metabolism. "When people eat hot chili, for instance, they often sweat, which is a sure sign of an increased metabolic rate," says Dr. Kenney. "The faster this rate, the more heat your body produces. And whatever warms you up slims you down."

So stock up on hot peppers, horseradish, chili powder and other spicy condiments, and use them often—especially in place of salt, which prompts some people to eat more than normal, says Dr. Kenney.

6. Feast on fiber. Fibrous foods often require thorough chewing, which slows down your eating. And eating more slowly usually means eating less, because your body has more time to recognize that it has received ample fuel. In addition, high-fiber foods tend to pack few calories per bite and, again, take up lots of room in the stomach.

Soluble fiber, best known for its cholesterol-cutting abilities, also depresses your body's insulin response—and your appetite. Normally, insulin levels rise after a meal, but soluble fiber keeps postmeal insulin levels lower, says Dr. Kenney, prompting your body to store less fat and crave less food.

Despite these many benefits, Americans consume only 12 to 15 grams of fiber daily, falling far short of the 25-gram recommendation. So stock up on barley, oat products,

Riding the Wave

Once the word *chocolate* weasels its way into your brain, it elbows aside every other thought until you can think of nothing else. Surrender is inevitable, right?

Wrong. Although we interpret cravings as commands, they're not. "People believe that cravings keep getting stronger until they finally have to give in," says Linda Crawford, M.D., an eating behavior specialist at Green Mountain at Fox Run, a residential weight- and health-management center for women in Ludlow, Vermont. But cravings will subside with time.

Research conducted at the University of Washington in Seattle shows that cravings follow wave patterns, starting and escalating, then peaking and subsiding. "Once you know for certain that a craving will decline, you can imagine yourself as a surfer," says Dr. Crawford, "riding the wave until it vanishes."

Just how long a ride are you in for? About 20 minutes. In the interim, engage in an activity that precludes eating—a walk, perhaps, an errand or a bike ride—then re-evaluate your hankerings. Decide rationally what, if anything, you crave and how much you'll eat. "The more you practice," promises Dr. Crawford, "the easier it becomes."

beans, apples, citrus fruits and root vegetables such as beets, carrots and potatoes, all of which contain lots of soluble fiber, and munch on these foods every day. Avoid fiber supplements—some are fraudulent, and others, if overused, can lead to severe constipation.

7. Eat simply. Multicourse meals may be gastronomically pleasant, but they can lead to excessive eating. "Serving a wide variety of foods at one meal can cause you to eat more than you normally would," says Thomas A. Wadden, Ph.D., director of the weight and eating disorders program at the University of Pennsylvania in Philadelphia, "primarily because each food has its own satiety level." In other words, after you've had your fill of roast beef, you may still crave the macaroni and cheese. Even after you've stuffed yourself with bread, you may go for seconds of the spaghetti. And of course, it's nearly impossible to resist "just a taste" of the dessert.

Limit entrées and side dishes to one per meal. Better yet, opt for a one-pot meal your whole family can enjoy.

8. Out-exercise your appetite. Got the munchies? Take a walk, ride a bike or head for the gym. Exercise reduces your immediate appetite by controlling insulin levels in your bloodstream (steady, lower insulin levels depress the appetite) and by heating the body (few people can eat a lot after intense aerobic exercise).

In the long run, a regular exercise program increases your appetite. But that's okay: You need fuel to power your workouts, after all. And if you increase the amount of food you eat by munching on lots of carbohydrates, you will undoubtedly take in fewer calories than the number you burn off by exercising.

9. Ask yourself why you want to eat. "Eighty-five percent of my patients have psychological or emotional motives for overeating," says Dr. Simonson. "And one of the primary reasons for this is stress, which makes many peo-

Rocks in the Road

A monstrous appetite can be tricky to tame—especially when practices presumed to suppress appetite and promote weight loss end up accomplishing the opposite. Following are the two most important traps to avoid in the battle of the bulge.

1. Severe dieting or meal skipping. Few things can increase your appetite like a prolonged restrictive diet, says Maria Simonson, Sc.D., Ph.D., director of the Health, Weight and Stress Clinic at Johns Hopkins Medical Institutions in Baltimore. When your body is low on fuel, your appetite increases in an effort to prompt you to eat more. And of course, starvation feels like punishment. "So many people overeat after starving themselves because they want a reward," says Dr. Simonson.

Skipping meals can also nurture a monstrous appetite, notes C. Wayne Callaway, M.D., a clinical nutritionist at George Washington University Medical Center in Washington, D.C. "People who skip breakfast or lunch tend to binge after dinner," he says. "It's a common problem among chronic dieters."

When you skip meals, the blood sugar and glycogen your body uses as fuel drop to very low levels. This, in turn, signals the body to demand more food, which makes you hungrier than normal. The solution? Worry less about cutting calories and focus instead on eating low-fat, high-carbohydrate, high-fiber foods. They're less likely than fatty foods to be

ple crave soft, creamy comfort foods, such as mashed potatoes with plenty of butter or a milk-and-cookies snack. It's the 'Nothin' says lovin' like somethin' from the oven' syndrome."

stored as fat, and they'll increase your metabolic rate after meals.

2. Mixing fats and sweets. "They're a deadly combination," says Thomas A. Wadden, Ph.D., director of the weight and eating disorders program at the University of Pennsylvania in Philadelphia. Each by itself heightens appetite, and the two together boost it doubly.

"Eating sweets can lead to a big increase in the amount of sugar in the blood, which causes insulin levels to soar," explains Nori Geary, Ph.D., associate professor at the Cornell University Medical Center in White Plains, New York. "Insulin then stimulates the metabolism of sugars, and in some people, the result is a lower blood sugar level than they started with—and a bigger appetite."

When fat is added to the equation, insulin levels rise much higher than they do when you eat sweets alone, says James Kenney, R.D., Ph.D., a nutrition-research specialist at the Pritikin Longevity Center in Santa Monica, California. "So it's best to avoid high-fat, high-sugar foods entirely. Very few people can limit themselves to 'just one bite.' "

If you crave something sweet, opt for a hard candy or mint. "Most people can't eat that many hard candies," says Dr. Kenney. "It's when sugar is combined with fat, as in a chocolate bar, or when it's in liquid form, as in a soft drink, that you can consume a lot of sugar very quickly and overstimulate insulin production in your body."

If you habitually turn to food to soothe bad feelings, you must develop an alternative strategy to make yourself feel better, says Dr. Simonson. And this means confronting your problem, not feeding it. Antistress measures, from counsel-

Calorie Accountability

If you fudge the facts about your diet and fitness habits, your nose may not grow, but your thighs surely will—or so say researchers at St. Luke's–Roosevelt Hospital Center in New York City. Scientists there found that many people who claim that they can't lose weight actually eat more and exercise less then they say they do. As a result, they sabotage their own efforts.

Participants in the St. Luke's study included 10 diet-resistant people and 80 successful losers, all of whom kept diaries in which they recorded their daily food intake and physical activity sessions. Researchers then compared the subjects' reported eating and exercising habits with their written claims and determined that the unsuccessful dieters actually ate twice as much and exercised only half as much as they told the researchers they did.

The moral of this story? Before you blame your weight on genetics or a low metabolism, make sure you know just how much you're eating and exactly how much you're moving. Guesses—even honest ones—don't count.

To help you hone your calorie-counting skills, check out *The Complete Brand-Name Guide to Choosing the Lowest Fat, Calorie, Cholesterol and Sodium Foods* by Densie Webb, R.D., Ph.D. This paperback is as jam-packed as its title, providing nutrient information for more than 2,000 name-brand products and including updates on labeling laws, tips for smart shopping and lists of guilt-free goodies you may not know about.

ing to yoga to a nice, hot bath, can also help you feel better and eat less.

10. Know your triggers. The smells, sights, sounds and even textures of foods are our most powerful incentives to eat—and to overeat. "Haven't we all eaten mediocre cookies just because they looked delicious?" Dr. Simonson asks. "Eating is so dependent on external cues that just seeing foods makes us want to eat." To eliminate the problem, simply bar fattening foods from the house. And if another member of the family must have sweets or high-fat foods on hand, ask him to hide the cache from you.

By keeping a regular food record, you can identify these kinds of cues. To start, set aside a half-hour a day for several days to write down everything you eat, why you ate it and why you started thinking about food. (Was it an advertisement? An emotion? An aroma?) Then look for patterns in your responses to certain stimuli. By identifying your appetite cues, you may be able to outsmart a craving the next time it rears its ugly head.

—Cathy Perlmutter

The Write Stuff

Frustrated by your attempt to lose weight? Set pen to paper, and vent some steam.

Rudyard Kipling referred to the written word as "the most powerful drug used by mankind." And the same can be said for the act of writing—especially if you write about yourself.

Because as the writer, you are the person for whom the written word is most enlightening, persuasive and powerful. You are the one for whom the act of writing about personal problems and situations may relieve stress and promote greater self-understanding. You, as the author of a personal journal, are the soul for whom writing can work miracles.

"The mind torments itself by thinking about unresolved issues," explains James Pennebaker, Ph.D., professor of psychology at Southern Methodist University in Dallas and author of *Opening Up: The Healing Power of Confiding in Others.* "A natural way to deal with these issues is to talk about them. But sometimes we just can't do that. The problems are too personal or too intimate, so we hold back. We worry. We obsess. And our inhibition creates stress."

The more we internalize external pressures, the more run-down our bodies become, and the more difficult it is to lose weight. We contract more colds, our blood pressure rises, and our heart rate accelerates. All because we haven't let off steam or, as Dr. Pennebaker suggests, unplugged our emotions and analyzed them by writing them down.

"When you write about a problem or experience, you start putting together all the thoughts that have been rattling around in your head," says Dr. Pennebaker. "The writing process organizes them into a coherent whole, which makes the problem less threatening. As a result, you're more likely to take action if need be."

And your body is less likely to take it on the chin. Why? Because you have a more effective immune system, says Dr. Pennebaker, who studied immune function in college freshmen participating in a four-day writing experiment. For 20 minutes each day, half of the students recorded their deepest feelings about a past trauma, while the rest wrote about objective experiences and situations. Blood samples were drawn before and after each writing session and again six weeks later.

The students who wrote about their emotions had higher blood concentrations of T-lymphocytes, a type of white blood cell that bolsters immune function, than the students who wrote about objective matters. And the effects lasted through the final blood test. Dr. Pennebaker also tracked the students' visits to the university health center. And as he suspected, the students who vented their emotions felt the need to visit the doctor fewer times than usual after writing about their problems.

Record Time

Convinced of the merits of writing but intimidated by the creative process? Relax, says Dr. Pennebaker. "Writing is a

Dear Diary

Tantalizing though the act may be, it's bad form to read someone else's diary—unless, of course, it has been published, like the journals listed below. Experience the threat of danger and the fever of passion as these women authors lived them, and allow their intimate accounts to inspire you to pen a few of your own.

Anne Frank: The Diary of a Young Girl. Anne Frank, a Jewish teenager, recounts her hopes and fears as she hides from the Nazis in Amsterdam during World War II. "I am grateful to God for giving me this gift of expressing all that is in me," writes Frank. "I can shake off everything if I write; my sorrows disappear, my courage is reborn."

Libby: The Sketches, Letters and Journals of Libby Beaman, 1879–1880. Beaman recounts her adventures as the first non–Native American woman to set foot on the Pribilot Islands, just outside the Arctic Circle. "All around me, I could hear the barking and hissing of the bulls," writes Beaman. " 'Seal mating is no sight a lady should have to witness,' one of the men said to me."

Henry and June: From the Unexpurgated Diary of Anaïs Nin. Anaïs Nin writes of her sexual awakening in 1932, the year she met Henry and June Miller. "The passivity of the woman's role weighs on me," writes Nin. "Rather than wait for his pleasure, I would like to take it, to run wild. Is it that which pushes me into lesbianism?"

Pioneer Women: Voices from the Kansas Frontier. Joanna F. Stratton compiles excerpts from the writings of many courageous women who helped settle the Great Plains. "A terrible storm and cloudburst came upon us, and we lost almost everything," writes Emma Mitchell New. "When we opened the door to get out, the water came up to our necks."

natural human activity; let nature take its course," he says. "After all, you don't have anything to lose. You don't have to be an Ernest Hemingway—or even an Erma Bombeck— for the process to work for you. We're not talking about a paper for English class or for publication; we're talking about a tool for personal insight."

Exactly. Keeping a journal isn't an academic exercise or a daily assignment. On the contrary, it's a simple, proven method for organizing your thoughts and understanding your feelings. And your words are for your eyes alone. No teachers. No criticism. No grades. Here's how to start.

Be your own guinea pig for three days. Find a quiet place where you won't be disturbed, and make it your writing room. Write for at least 15 minutes at a time for three consecutive days, and see how you like it. If you keep a daily food diary, elaborating on your regular entries may be the perfect way to start.

"Disclosing intimate parts of yourself may take some practice," says Dr. Pennebaker. "And if you've never written or talked about your thoughts and feelings, you may find it awkward at first. But give it time." If you find that you're stymied, try using a typewriter or computer instead of pen and paper, or talk into a tape recorder to begin.

Write continuously about issues, persons or events that are on your mind. Describe your experiences, and explore your feelings about them. Don't agonize over grammar, vocabulary or sentence structure. Just let the words flow.

Expect to feel sad or depressed immediately after writing. You're summoning up unpleasant feelings, after all. But any negativity will disappear in an hour or so, and in three to four days, your mood will lift again as you gain perspective about your current situation.

Keep your journal to yourself. "If you plan to show your writing to someone, subconsciously you will write for them," says Dr. Pennebaker. "When you are the only audience, you don't have to rationalize or justify yourself in your writing. As a result, your writing will be more honest and straightforward—and it will help you more."

Write for clarification and revelation, not as a substitute for action. "Writing works when you are angry, frustrated or distraught," says Dr. Pennebaker, "but you must take care not to become absorbed in the process. Writing should facilitate action, not replace it."

—Linda Miller

The Late Late Chow

Best and worst midnight snacks—how to fill up your tank without blowing your waistline.

It's 11:30 P.M., and without thinking, I've clicked the remote to NBC. Which is bad news. Because as the technicolor curtains part and Jay's head pops up on the screen, I can think of only one thing: those old Doritos commercials. The saliva flows, the cabinets call, and next thing, I've blown an entire day of reasonably disciplined eating in a single binge. Then I'm in bed, either restless with indigestion or wrestling with another nightmare: Instead of summoning delta waves, I'm being chased by Delta Burke wielding a spiced beef stick.

But while chips and salami aren't the best of snacks, that doesn't mean a person must be forced to ignore the rumblings of his stomach in the midnight hour. We've consulted the experts and come up with some of the best foods to satisfy you, foods that won't cut into your sleep or leave you stuffed. First, though, remember the six principles of nighttime eating.

Health-Food Impostors

Just because it's in health-food stores and ruddy-faced out-door types eat it, that doesn't mean it should be on your plate. Look beyond appearances and check out what's inside.

1. Granola. The majority of granolas on the market are loaded with fat, as much as 27 grams in a single serving. And that's without milk. "Traditional granolas are high in coconut oil, a saturated fat, and that's the worst kind for you," says Martin Yadrick, R.D., a nutritionist and spokesperson for the American Dietetic Association. There are low-fat varieties, but read the label before you indulge. Rule of thumb: If it has more than 2 grams of fat per serving, pass it by.

2. Bran muffins. Ever notice how some bran muffins leave your napkin and your hands greasy? That's from all the oil inside. A typical small bran muffin contains 4 grams of fat, and some large ones may have as much as 12 grams and 900 calories. Opting for a bagel gets you down to 1.4 grams of fat and 160 calories.

1. Don't have a cow. Meats and other high-protein foods are a mistake before bed. Protein supplies the brain with the amino acid tyrosine, which boosts alertness. "This is the last thing you want when you're trying to sleep," says Judith Wurtman, Ph.D., nutrition researcher in the Department of Brain and Cognitive Science at the Massachusetts Institute of Technology in Cambridge. Foods high in protein also tend to be high in fat, which digests slowly and makes sleep more fitful. So think twice before grabbing for that cold roast beef, not to mention the Cheddar, fontina or Swiss cheese.

2. Break bread before bed. Your body starts processing

3. Apple juice. Apples are a terrific source of vitamin C and fiber. But apple juice is little more than sugar water. You're better off with a glass of cranberry juice, which is loaded with vitamin C.

4. Frozen yogurt. Some brands of frozen yogurt contain up to seven grams of fat per serving. Read the label, and don't take home any brand with more than three grams of fat per serving. Try Colombo nonfat yogurt, I Can't Believe It's Yogurt! nonfat and TCBY's nonfat flavors.

5. Carob. Carob candy won't save you from the sins of chocolate. Both contain virtually the same amount of fat, and at least chocolate doesn't taste like rabbit pellets.

6. Trail mix. It's fine to munch on nuts, seeds and dried fruit for energy during a ten-mile hike, but don't eat handfuls of the stuff at home. The seeds and nuts are loaded with fat, and the dried fruit contains lots of calories. Fresh fruit and pretzels are better snacks.

carbohydrates—foods such as rice, potatoes and breads—immediately. Furthermore, they help speed tryptophan, a sleep-inducing amino acid, to the brain. "Diets that don't contain enough carbohydrates usually turn people into insomniacs," says Dr. Wurtman.

3. Watch for hidden caffeine. Most of us know not to down five cups of coffee before sleeping, but insidious caffeine sources abound. An 8-ounce cup of tea and a 12-ounce can of cola both contain around 35 milligrams of caffeine, about equal to a 4-ounce cup of instant coffee. Many drugstore decongestants and nonprescription painkillers also include caffeine. Two tablets of regular-strength Anacin, for cxample, have 64 milligrams. Beware of chocolate as well; if you're craving it, try some hot chocolate, which has only 4 milligrams of caffeine.

4. Doff the nightcap. Booze may help you fall asleep, but alcohol disrupts your rest by reducing deep sleep and dream sleep, the phases of sleep that leave you refreshed.

5. Avoid the heat in the night. Spicy foods can generate a lot of stomach acid; when you're lying down, the acid can easily back up into the lower esophagus and cause heartburn—and nightmares. "You may feel as though you're being stabbed with an ice pick, when in fact it's just the pepperoni you ate," says Dr. Wurtman. Either that or you've seen *Basic Instinct* too many times.

6. Banish bedtime binges. Finally, if you're an incorrigible midnight gourmand, here's an incentive to hold the line against overindulging. Many experts believe that food eaten at night has more of a chance of being stored as body fat than the same food eaten in the daytime. This is likely because there are fewer bodily functions occurring while you sleep that require energy, explains James O. Hill, Ph.D., associate director of the Center for Human Nutrition at the University of Colorado Health Sciences Center in Denver. The net result: "More of the food you're eating is going into storage," he says.

Best Midnight Snacks

After-hours noshing doesn't have to be a disaster. With some foresight, you can have tasty, filling, healthy foods ready to go.

English muffin pizza. Start by cracking open an English muffin, then spoon on tomato sauce and sprinkle it all with a couple of tablespoons of grated low-fat mozzarella. (You can add a pinch of oregano if you want to get fancy.)

Throw your contraption in the toaster oven or run it under the broiler for a few minutes. All told, this snack is under 400 calories, with less than ten grams of fat. That's less than half the fat in two slices of pepperoni pizza from Pizza Hut.

Another option is to check out the frozen-food section of your supermarket. Someone's figured out how to make low-fat versions of pizza that still taste pretty good. We like Weight Watchers pepperoni pizza and Stouffer's Lean Cuisine French bread pizzas. Neither brand contains more than 350 calories or 11 grams of fat.

Turkey breast sandwiches. Talk about sandwiches, and the mind turns to Dagwood, a man well-attuned to his instincts though, as a consequence, perhaps not a pillar of self-control. The fact is, a sandwich can be a sensible snack. Two ounces of turkey breast is nearly 13 times less fattening than the same amount of beef salami. Other good sandwich fillers include lean roast beef, grilled chicken cutlet or any kind of nonbreaded fish. In the shrink-wrapped deli category, Healthy Choice makes a good thin-sliced cooked ham (about one-half gram of fat per three-slice serving) and turkey breast (about one gram of fat per three slices).

As a reward for going light on the filling, treat yourself to a good, hearty bread, such as whole-grain, pita or French bread—any kind is high in carbohydrates and low in fat. But go easy on the toppings, which can blow your whole day's fat budget in a single swipe. Best bets: reduced-calorie or fat-free mayonnaise, low-fat or fat-free salad dressing and as much lettuce, tomatoes and mushrooms as you want.

Wait, you say you need cheese, too? Okay, but choose low-fat versions and keep the portions light. Borden makes excellent low-fat American, Cheddar, mozzarella and Swiss cheeses, all with 35 calories and two grams of fat per slice.

Sundaes. If you're in the mood for ice cream, instead go for nonfat frozen yogurt or sherbet for ten grams of fat savings over premium ice cream. Top it with all the fruit you want—sliced banana, blackberries or strawberries—but hold off on the nuts. Finally, pour on some Estee ChocoSyp, a chocolate syrup with no fat and only 20 calories per tablespoon. Some frozen yogurts we like include Häagen-Dazs low-fat, TCBY nonfat flavors and Yoplait low-fat vanilla orange cremes (ice pops). American Glace also makes a good fat-free frozen dessert. Have to have ice cream? Try one of the new fat-free kinds, such as Sealtest's, which is delicious.

Cereals. Breakfast cereal makes one of the best midnight snacks. Cornflakes are only 100 calories per cup and have no fat. Most any of the other cereals will do just as well, and if you're smart enough to use skim milk, you almost can't go wrong. For those who love granola, check out Kellogg's Low Fat Granola, which has whole oats and wheat but no cholesterol and less than half the fat (two grams) of the other granolas.

Cheese-flavored popcorn. Start with air-popped popcorn and add a shake of grated Parmesan or Romano cheese. Total fat content: 2.1 grams. Other flavorings to experiment with include chopped dates, raisins or cinnamon. Among commercial varieties, check out Boston Lite's Gourmet Popcorn (3 grams of fat) or Weight Watchers White Cheddar Cheese Popcorn (4 grams of fat).

Pretzels. These offer a great low-fat, low-sodium alternative to chips. Wege markets an excellent variety made from natural sourdough bread (less than a gram of fat per serving). But if you're an avowed chip fan, try the no-oil baked tortilla chip from Guiltless Gourmet, which has 1.5 grams of fat per serving. The company also makes an excellent barbecue pinto bean dip.

Baked goods. Snack Well's Fat Free Devil's Food Cookie Cakes are a fine example of the trend to low- and nonfat desserts. More good baked goods: Entenmann's Fat-Free Chocolate Crunch Cake and Weight Watchers (frozen) Double Fudge Cake.

Low-fat cookies. We like Entenmann's Oatmeal Raisin Cookies. At only 80 calories for every two, with no fat, these are a fine choice for cookie-munchers. Another kind we like is R.W. Frookies apple spice cookies—also with no fat. Or steal your kid's animal crackers; 13 of them can have fewer than two grams of fat. Other good grocery buys include Sunshine Golden Fruit Raisin Biscuits and Pepperidge Farm Wholesome Choice carrot walnut cookies.

Snack bars. Try the Sunsweet California Prune and Almond Bar. More nutritious than an Almond Joy any night, this fruit and nut bar is lightly coated with chocolate, so there's only a moderate amount of fat (six grams). Other high-carbohydrate, low-fat "sports bars" are also great at night. Some of these take a little getting used to, but we like PowerBar's Wild Berry, the citrus-flavored Edgebar and the oat bran–flavored Exceed sports bar. For those craving peanut butter, which is normally loaded with fat, Fi-Bar makes a vanilla peanut butter crunch snack bar with four grams of fat—one-fourth of what you'd get in two tablespoons of peanut butter.

Licorice. Twizzlers and other licorice-type candies are good nonfat alternatives to candy bars. Other good ways to satisfy your craving for sweets without getting any fat: hard candies, gummy bears, jelly beans.

Fruit with cottage cheese. One cup of blackberries contains loads of fiber and half the daily requirement of vitamin C, plus they're low in calories, sodium, cholesterol and fat. Combine them with low-fat cottage cheese, and you have a snack under 160 calories. Sliced pears, apples and apricots are equally good as toppings, as are dried fruits.

—David Zinczenko

Part Six

Use Muscle-Building to Banish Fat

Muscle Your Way to Weight Loss

*Use Dr. Wayne Westcott's body-shaping plan to tone
and trim a new you.*

You remember dieting—that torturous activity
we've all, at one time, put ourselves through to get
flatter tummies, firmer legs and thinner thighs. Like
carbon paper, the eight-track tape and the dreaded
leisure suit (you remember yours), dieting has become obsolete. It's been replaced by a better, simpler way to achieve results that stay around forever.

That simpler way no doubt involves a healthy eating regimen of low-fat foods—all becoming more
and more plentiful in our supermarkets each day. But
it also relies on exercise, a remedy-in-motion that not
only reduces risk for a variety of illnesses but also
skims off flab, tones bellies and slims down hips.

Exercise, you say? What else is new? Lots. *Prevention* magazine's fitness advisor Wayne Westcott,
Ph.D., national strength consultant for the YMCA
and the National Academy of Sports Medicine, has
laid out the exercise formula to get the job done.
He's used it at his gym, conducting studies with
hundreds of participants—with dramatic results.

Dramatic results, but by simple means. The time put in each week by Dr. Westcott's subjects amounted to no more than the time it takes to watch a made-for-TV movie. In roughly 80 minutes per week for eight weeks, the folks in this program saw results dieting alone could never offer. Read on for the whys and hows.

The Key Isn't Just Motion—It's Muscle, Too

Aside from being a miserable activity, dieting is also mean-spirited. It steals away the very material you need to excuse yourself from ever having to diet again. We call that stuff muscle, the weight your body can't afford to lose.

"The scale tells you how much less you weigh without telling you what you really lost, which is fat and muscle," says Dr. Westcott. "Muscle is so important in so many things we do throughout the day—you can't afford to lose it." Plus, because muscle devours calories more hungrily than fat tissue can, the more of it you have, the less likely your body needs to diet.

Now, you don't need to be on a diet to lose muscle; just being inactive can sap the hard stuff from your body. The typical sedentary American loses an average of 5 pounds of the hard stuff each decade—while gaining 15 pounds of fat at the same time. "On a bathroom scale, that would indicate a 10-pound weight-gain problem (15 fat pounds minus 5 muscle pounds)," says Dr. Westcott. "But the reality is that it's actually a 20-pound problem (15 pounds more fat plus 5 pounds less muscle)."

This situation sends you on a bullet train to Blobville, as increasing muscle loss slows your metabolic rate, or your body's calorie-burning engine. This makes it even more difficult to maintain a healthy weight, as your sluggish furnace allows more body fat to gather. "Overall body composition,

(continued on page 162)

Dr. Westcott's Body-Shaper Program

Bench press. This compound exercise builds and strengthens the chest muscles, triceps of the upper arms and upper latissimus dorsi muscles (lats) of your back. Lie on an exercise bench, with your knees bent and your feet flat on the floor and shoulder-width apart. Grasp dumbbells or a barbell with your hands slightly more than just shoulder-width apart. Slowly lower the weight to your chest. The weight should not actually touch it. Press the weight up until arms are fully extended, with elbows almost locked. Repeat.

Leg press. This compound exercise focuses on the quadriceps, hamstrings, buttocks and calves. Sit on a leg-press machine, place your feet on the resistance plate and press out until your legs are straight. Bend your knees and let the weights return to the original starting point. Repeat.

Seated pulley row. This exercise helps work the lats, rhomboids (upper back), brachialis (upper arms), deltoids (shoulders), biceps and forearms as well as the trapezius, which is the largest muscle of the back and neck, and erector muscles, which support the spine. Sit on the machine with your knees slightly flexed. Your feet should be up against an object to maintain stability. Keep your upper torso erect and your lower back flexed. Grip the handle and pull it slowly and smoothly to your upper abdomen. As you pull in, keep your arms close to your sides. Try not to use your torso to pull the weight. Return to the starting position, with the weights going back down. Repeat.

Seated quadriceps extension. This exercise focuses on the quadriceps. Sit with the base of your shins against the inner side of the padded resistance bar. Push the bar forward and upward until your legs are straight. Don't swing the legs up fast—do it slowly and with control. Then, allow your legs to return to starting position. If your knees hurt or it's too difficult to go to the full extension, just do a partial repetition, shortening the path. (Use ankle weights if you don't have an extension machine.)

Hamstring curl. Lie facedown, with your heels under the padded resistance bar, holding on to the front of the leg-curl machine. Curl your legs up until your calves touch the upper part of your thighs. Return to the down position and repeat. If you don't have a leg-curl machine, a partner can help provide some resistance against your legs.

Lat machine pull-down. This compound exercise targets the upper back, biceps, forearm flexors and brachialis muscles. Stand facing the lat machine, reach up and take an overhand grip on the bar, with your hands set three to five inches wider than your shoulders. Straighten your arms and use your weight to pull your body downward, and then wedge your knees under the restraint. Allow the weights to pull your shoulders upward to stretch your lats. Use your upper back and arms to pull the bar down to touch behind the neck. Hold this for a moment and then return slowly to the starting position.

Overhead press. This compound exercise (also known as the military press) works the deltoids, triceps and upper back muscles. Raise the weight to shoulder height. Sit with your feet firmly on the floor. Keeping your back straight, slowly press the bar to arm's length overhead, pause, then lower. Don't bounce the weight off your chest. Repeat. This can be done with free weights or on a machine.

Biceps curl. This exercise targets the biceps but also gives some work to the brachialis muscles and forearm flexors. Hold a barbell with both hands, palms facing up. Stand with your back straight, with the bar at arm's length against your

(continued)

Dr. Westcott's Body-Shaper Program—
Continued

upper thighs. Curl the bar up in a semicircular motion until your forearms touch your biceps. Keep your upper arms and elbows close to the sides of your body. Lower the bar slowly to the starting position using the same path. Repeat.

Triceps extension. This exercise targets the triceps. While sitting with your feet firmly on the floor, hold a dumbbell with both hands overhead at arm's length. Lower the weight behind your head in a semicircular motion until your forearms touch your biceps. Return to an overhead position using the same path. Repeat.

Triceps push-down. Stand in front of the lat machine and grasp the bar, palms down. Start with forearms and biceps touching. Press the bar down in a semicircular motion until your arms are extended. Return slowly to the starting position. While you're doing this, try your best to keep your abdominal muscles tense.

Lower back exercise. Position the front of your upper body over the end of a waist-high bench. Bend over with your head down and your hands placed lightly behind your

not just body weight, should be stressed," says Dr. Westcott. Manipulating body composition means not just watching fatty foods and taking brisk walks but also upping your muscle activity.

The 20–20 solution. Dr. Westcott proved this point in an eight-week study reported at the IDEA World Research Forum, a meeting of fitness professionals from 60 countries held last year in New Orleans. He took a group of average Joes and Josephines and put them through a program using both resistance and aerobic exercise—showing how easy it ears. Slowly raise your torso until you're level with the bench. Repeat.

Neck exercise. Sit on a bench with your back straight, head up. Place both hands on your forehead. Push your head back as far as comfortable while resisting with your neck muscles. Use only moderate resistance. Do ten repetitions. Then place your hands on the back of your head and repeat the movement in reverse.

Sit-back. This exercise really targets your abdominal muscles. While sitting tilted back at a 45-degree angle on a mat, with knees bent and your hands across your chest, lower yourself all the way down to a count of ten. Uncross your hands, turn onto your elbow and push yourself up again; then do another. Try a set of six for starters; add a repetition or two as they get easier.

Abdominal curl. Lie on your back with your knees bent, fingers lightly touching your ears. You can place your hands behind your head as long as you don't use them to pull your head forward. Slowly curl your upper torso only until your shoulders leave the floor. Hold for a few seconds, go down and repeat, inhaling as you go down. If this is too difficult, keep your arms at your sides.

can be to rework your body composition for the better.

During the program, 282 adults performed 20 minutes of muscle strengthening, along with 20 minutes of aerobic exercise, two or three days a week. That's all. Sure, some may have added extra walking on the weekend. The bottom line: The folks who worked out for just 80 minutes a week over eight weeks saw great results.

The average fat loss was 8½ pounds (a little over a pound a week—a healthy pace, say most experts), with an accompanying burst of a 3-pound muscle gain. That translates into a mean body composition improvement of 11½ pounds (8½ plus 3) in just eight weeks!

Now, if you were simply out to lose weight, you'd be pretty miffed. After all, if you weren't hitting the weights, you'd be three pounds lighter. But you'd also be weaker, less toned, less fit and, all in all, not as healthy without that extra muscle. It's the stuff needed to maintain basic daily functions as you grow older. A street gang of age-related degenerative processes arrives largely because of muscle loss and its impact on function.

"Your muscle is like an engine, and losing it is like going from a six- to a four- to a two-cylinder car," says Dr. Westcott. "Soon you can't go up even small hills anymore when you used to be able to go up mountains!" With that in mind, it's no wonder each increase in muscle expands your boundaries of daily activity.

Not only that, but more muscle means a firmer, shapelier body as well. Of course, improving function and metabolism is nice, but looking good isn't so bad either.

Results go interior. Dr. Westcott's research also supports previous strength-training studies, suggesting that the benefits of this program aren't limited strictly to slimmer waistlines and better function. "We are also seeing significant blood pressure reductions in some of the older folks," says Dr. Westcott. In fact, the workouts have done such a number on high blood pressure in a few people that they actually decreased or eliminated their use of medications.

"We also have reports of participants with adult-onset diabetes responding quite favorably as they increase muscle mass," says Dr. Westcott. No surprise—increased muscle mass and activity help out by burning more glucose, which is running wild because the insulin isn't taking effect. "With that in mind, strong muscles should prove a major aspect of preventive medicine and rehabilitation," says Dr. Westcott.

Other, more immediate benefits also occurred for the

older people who entered the study at ground zero in terms of fitness. Some folks coming in with canes or walkers finished the program without them. "Many of the participants are able to do things on their own that they couldn't do before," says Dr. Westcott. This is especially true in seniors where quadriceps (front thigh muscle) strength is critical in getting up and out of chairs and cars and going up stairs. The leg exercises used in this program help combat that weakness.

The Body-Shaping Recipe

Now, reporting these findings is fine, but wouldn't it be better to have the actual blueprint for these benefits in hand?

The complete program boils down to two to three aerobic sessions and two to three strength-training sessions, each lasting approximately 20 minutes. It's up to you how you'd like to spread it out over the week. For example, you may want to work out three times a week, with the strength

Hands Off

According to research conducted at the University of Wisconsin–La Crosse, you burn more calories on the stair-climber when you swing your arms than when you grasp the handrails.

Fifteen women and 15 men tackled three stair-climbing strategies: standing upright, leaning forward onto the console and standing upright while using the handrails for support. The results? Standing tall with hands off the rails provided a more challenging (and calorie-burning) workout for everyone.

and aerobic components done together—or you may want to have one workout each day for a six-day cycle. Keep in mind, however, that you don't want to strength-train the same muscles two days in a row, because those muscles need time to regroup and repair to get stronger. Here are the two elements you need.

Go aerobic. In Dr. Westcott's plan, participants chose from treadmill walking, bench stepping and stationary cycling. Basically, though, any sustained aerobic activity you enjoy will do fine. If you're going to do your aerobics and strength-training on the same day, it really doesn't matter which one you do first.

"We have found that improvements are the same no matter what you do first," says Dr. Westcott. Of course, it always helps to include a warm-up session before and a cooldown after exercise—just a few minutes of walking or easy jogging should be enough. Once you do get going into your 20-minute session, aim for an exertion level that gets you sweating but still allows you to talk without feeling winded.

Muscle up. Dr. Westcott chose the strength exercises in this chapter for two reasons: (1) They're highly efficient, hitting all the major muscle groups, and (2) they come as close as possible to mimicking your daily activities, so you can do those activities more effectively.

"Compound exercises, such as leg presses, bench presses and rows, involve several muscle groups at the same time," says Dr. Westcott. "These are more useful than other exercises in terms of function because they use movements similar to what we do in normal life—that is, all the pushing and pulling."

The workout also includes simpler moves, such as leg extensions, arm curls and trunk curls. "You might want to just start out with the three compound exercises mentioned earlier. By so doing, you have worked almost all your major muscle groups in a very functional manner," says Dr. Westcott. "Progress from there as you become stronger, working in the other exercises, like the lower back and neck exercises, which really help the vertebral column," says Dr. Westcott.

The most astounding thing about the program is not just the modest amount of time needed but also the volume of exercise required. Dr. Westcott included 11 weight-training exercises in his program. But the participants performed only one set, doing 8 to 12 repetitions in each, during each workout. For your own muscles, find a weight or resistance level that you feel comfortable doing for your single set at those repetitions. By the last few repetitions, the exercise should feel pretty tough but still doable. After a few weeks, when the exercise gets easy, kick up the resistance a bit or do more repetitions to make it more challenging. "It helps to work the large muscle groups first and move down to the smaller ones," says Dr. Westcott. That way you won't tire the small muscles first, hindering the larger exercises.

—Greg Gutfeld

Workouts That Work!

Surefire ways to muscle-up your metabolism and lose weight without dieting.

At a recent *Prevention* magazine Health and Fitness Festival, we had the pleasure of meeting many readers who have turned to lifting weights to bolster their walking programs for a total-body workout.

One question kept coming up over and over, however: "With the very limited amount of free time I have in my schedule, can I really do enough strength-training to benefit my body?"

The answer is simple. Yes, you can get stronger, firmer and shapelier without spending hours in your gym shorts. As long as you hit the muscles the right way—with the right exercises, the right number of sets and the proper amount of rest—you can get great results in minutes. That's right, minutes—30 of 'em, to be exact.

Less Is More (more or less)

You have hundreds of muscles in your body. Some help you get your luggage off a rack; others help you blink an eyelid. The key in training is to narrow the field.

You want to target the biggies—the major muscle groups. But to do it in less time, you want to hit them in bunches. And to do that you need compound exercises.

A compound exercise combines movements that work more than one muscle at the same time. A leg press, for example, hits the quadriceps (the muscles on the front of your thighs), hamstrings (the muscles on the back of your thighs) and buttocks as well as the calves of the lower legs. "Essentially, with a leg press or similar compound exercise, you're doing four exercises in one," says exercise physiologist and physical therapist Phil Dunphy, director of Hudson Physical Therapy in Jersey City, New Jersey.

By doing compound exercises like the bench press, military press and leg press, you avoid doing specific exercises that cover less territory but eat up more time. You get the same results with time to spare. (See "Dr. Westcott's Body-Shaper Program" on page 160.)

Order equals speed. To keep your workout short and to the point, get yourself in order.

"By alternating upper-body exercises with lower-body ones, you don't tire as quickly, and you don't need to rest as much," says Doug Semenick, certified strength and conditioning specialist and director of the wellness program at the University of Louisville in Kentucky. If you must do upper-body exercises in a straight sequence, then alternate the pushing ones with the pulling ones.

With the bench press, for example, you push the weight up; with the lat pull-down (works the latissimus dorsi, a back muscle), you pull the weight toward you. Each exercise works an opposing, or antagonistic, muscle group. Do those one after the other, and tired muscles won't slow you down. And you shave minutes of rest off your workout.

If you have time to do exercises that work smaller muscles as well as those that work big muscles, start with the biggies first.

"How Hard Should I Push Myself?"

A question readers frequently ask regards intensity. "How should the exercise feel when I'm doing it? Should I be grunting and groaning to near exhaustion, or should I pick a weight level that offers little resistance at all? How do I know where to start?"

Ideally, you should try to do sets of 8 to 10 repetitions at about 75 percent of your 1-repetition maximum (the amount of weight you can lift in one shot). That means if you can lift 100 pounds once in a given exercise, then your sets should be at around 75 pounds, to be done for 8 to 10 repetitions. Once the tenth rep becomes easy, you move up. (Wait a workout or two before moving up, and increase the repetitions to 11 or 12 in the meantime, just to be on the safe side.)

To find the right intensity, you don't really have to find how much you do at one repetition. Instead, simply start out with a light weight and feel your way up the ladder. Once you find a resistance in which ten repetitions are kind of tough to do, you're probably near or at that 75 percent range. Stay there until it gets easy. You can even start out at a lighter level anyway. That just gets you prepared for tougher sets down the road.

The reason for exercising at this level of intensity has to do with the makeup of the muscle. Muscle is made of fibers, which respond to stress. Research and anecdotal evidence suggest that the level of intensity mentioned above is what's needed to stimulate muscle growth and strength.

The reason for this is simple: Smaller muscles tire faster, and if you do them before the larger muscles, they'll fail on you. "If you went to do an arm-and-back exercise but you already exercised your forearms, for example, then that smaller area of muscle may be too tired to hold the bar and keep a strong-enough grip throughout the exercise," says Semenick.

Put the small stuff that isolates the smaller muscles at or near the end of the workout. Given limited time, you get the most bang for your buck by working the larger muscles. And if you plan on doing lower back, neck or abdominal exercises, hold them off till the very end, too. You may bog down if you start with them.

For proof, you can try this experiment (or maybe just think about trying it). Do as many partial sit-ups as you can—safely—in two minutes. Then turn over and try a couple of push-ups. "Your belly should flop to the floor," says Semenick. Sit-ups nail your upper and lower body's stabilizer muscles, so once they're taxed, your body becomes unable to perform any other total-body exercise with any real force.

If you are in a big hurry and would rather skip abdominal exercises, you can sneak them in when you're doing other exercises. "By tensing up your abdominal muscles when you're doing a triceps push-down, for example, you're working those muscles effectively," says Dunphy. "And when you're doing pull-ups, all you really have to do is think about your abdominals, and they're getting worked." By concentrating on them as you pull up and let yourself down, your body's on automatic pilot, tensing those muscles every step of the way.

The rightful rest. Rest is vital, but you don't need a siesta. When you're exercising a muscle, you're working through its "energy system," which is really no more than the muscle's gas tank. In the time it takes to do those crucial eight to ten repetitions, you've sapped the muscle's immediate energy source of fuel—now it needs a nap to get it back to full power. "Temporary muscle failure drains all the energy the muscle has stored in it," says Semenick. Rest for 30 seconds, and you've recovered half of it. In one minute, you've recovered roughly 75 percent. After two minutes, nearly all—or 94 percent—is recovered.

"You shouldn't have to wait any more than that to get back into the next set with adequate strength and power," says Semenick.

You can rest two minutes between heavy sets of the same exercise, but you can probably shorten or eliminate the rest when you change from one exercise to a new one that works different muscles. You may have to rest only a minute or less between a leg press and a bench press, for example, since the former targets the legs and the latter hits the chest.

Two Sets and You're Set

Remember that you perform exercises in sets, which are groups of repetitions done successively, with rest in between each group. The key is to do enough but not go overboard. But how many is enough?

When you're lifting weights, you're constantly breaking down muscle that is later rebuilt with a bonus. One powerful set hits the muscle hard. Another set repeats the process but to a lesser degree, as your muscles fatigue more. Same for a third set.

As you go on, improvements in both strength and muscle mass will get smaller and smaller. "The number of sets begins to mean very little," says James Graves, Ph.D., chair of the health and physical education department at Syracuse University in New York. "If you exercise to momentary fatigue or muscle exhaustion, you have used most fibers in the muscle. That's really what you want." You can do that—believe it or not—in just one or two sets.

"By trial and error, researchers and athletes have found

that once you've depleted the energy from the muscle and tired it out, the extra sets aren't worth the time required to complete them," says Dr. Graves.

The law of diminishing returns starts coming into play— "unless, of course, the participant has specific goals related to muscle size and endurance," he says.

Less, therefore, may mean more. As long as you push your muscles to fatigue—where you can barely lift the weight at the last repetition—you've done the job.

Settle on one or two sets per exercise. After that—by doing three, four or more—you aren't substantially upping the load as much as you did with that increase from one to two sets.

In each set, do your repetitions in a slow, controlled fashion, concentrating on the movement. Make it last roughly six seconds—two for the phase when you're bringing the weight up (called the concentric phase) and four for the phase when you're letting the weight down (called the eccentric phase). By doing this with a reasonable weight, you tire the muscle fully.

By doing more sets with a minimum rest interval, you may be building endurance, but further improvements in muscular strength are minimal. "You get infinitely more out of doing a few slow sets than you get by doing six sets real fast and sloppy," says Dunphy.

Think about it—two sets of ten repetitions at six seconds a pop. Throw a two-minute rest between the sets, and you have four minutes total for the muscle group. Not much, eh?

The same goes for abdominal exercises. Many folks feel the need to spend hours on that section of flesh, when only a handful of repetitions will do. Don't do 1,000 abs—do 20 slow, hard ones.

"Eccentric sit-ups—when you stress the movement slowly on the way down—are a perfect example of an exercise that creates full intensity with very few reps needed," says Dunphy. "You can do all the reps and sets in the world, but without the tension brought on by the eccentric phase, forget it."

Aim for a full repetition every time. When you can't do most of your full range of motion in any exercise while keeping the weight under control, it's time to quit. And remember, if you're just beginning, don't knock yourself out. Get your body used to lifting weights by using light amounts and going slow. As you get comfortable with the exercises, then you can start pushing yourself a little harder. At that point, you should exercise with a partner—someone who can monitor you (and you them) in case the weight is more than you can handle.

Two Workouts That Work

Strength-training workouts can last two or three hours, and you may spend only minutes actually doing any real work. We're out to change that. Below is a program that incorporates all the tips from above. We're talking total work, no waste—hitting all the major muscle groups with enough rest time in between. And it adds up to 30 minutes flat.

If you want a little more mass, or you just want to spice things up and you have extra time, we've added specific exercises to push the time commitment up to 45 minutes.

You can mix and match these workouts, too. For example, during the week, you can do the short program twice and then reserve one longer workout as "the weekender"—something to do on a Saturday or Sunday when you have more time to spare.

Or if you plan on working out just twice a week (which is the minimum prescription from the American College of Sports Medicine), you can alternate one with the other. Remember to take it slow, and check with your doctor if you have any medical conditions that may interfere with exercise.

30-Minute Flex

- 2 sets of leg presses—1 minute per set with 2 minutes rest between sets; 1 minute rest between last set and next exercise: bench press.
- 2 sets of bench presses—1 minute per set with 2 minutes rest between sets; 2 minutes rest between bench press and next exercise: rows.
- 2 sets of rows—1 minute per set with 2 minutes rest between sets; 2 minutes rest between last row and next exercise: military press.
- 2 sets of military presses—1 minute per set with 2 minutes rest between sets; 2 minutes rest between last set and next exercise: lat pull-downs.
- 2 sets of lat pull-downs—1 minute per set with 2 minutes rest between sets; 1 minute rest between last set and next exercise: abdominals.
- 1 set of abdominals—2 minutes.

All done!

Total time: 12 minutes of exercise + 18 minutes of rest = 30 minutes flat.

45 Minutes for Extra Tone

If you have the time to sink your teeth into a meatier workout, try this one on for size. Just do the same as above, but continue on with one minute of rest between abdominals and the next exercise: biceps curls.

- 2 sets of biceps curls—1 minute per set with 2 minutes rest between sets; 1 minute rest between last set and next exercise: leg extension.

• 2 sets of leg extensions—1 minute per set with 2 minutes rest between sets; 1 minute of rest between last set and next exercise: triceps push-down.

• 2 sets of triceps push-downs—1 minute per set with 2 minutes rest between sets.

Total time: 30 minutes of first workout + 6 minutes of new exercises + 9 minutes of rest = 45 minutes flat.

—Greg Gutfeld

The Deskside Stretch

Unknot tension-tied muscles with these eight easy stretches.

There's no doubt that sitting at a desk all day can result in poor circulation, tight muscles and stiff, aching joints. Add to that the posture and wrist problems associated with staring at a computer screen or typing for hours at a time and the poor design of most workstations, and you've got a major problem—your body is sluggish, and your mind, barely there.

How can you ease the tension and regain alertness? Stretch, and stretch again, suggests nationally renowned flexibility trainer and consultant Bob Anderson. These eight sitting and standing moves can be done at your desk. Use them several times a day to keep from becoming a "working stiff."

Sitting

Hand release. For hands and fingers. With your palms facing down, separate and straighten your fingers until the tension of a stretch is felt. Hold for

Weights Can Shatter Bad Body Image

When the mirror shows you a body you don't like, don't reach for another diet. Reach for the barbells instead. A new study shows that resistance-training can help you shed those bad feelings about your body—without losing weight. For the first time, researchers targeted the body images of middle-aged women, asking 60 of them to rate how they felt about things like their posture, tone of their abdomens, waist size, body profile and body weight. Then the women embarked on a three-times-a-week program of either walking or resistance-training. When they rated themselves three months later, the weight lifters' body images had improved nearly twice as much as the walkers'. What's more, their body images jumped even though neither group lost a pound.

Resistance-training may have the corner on body-image building because its effects are readily visible, says study author Larry A. Tucker, Ph.D., professor and director of health promotion at Brigham Young University in Provo, Utah. "It's one of the very few natural ways you can change the way you look." You also get a boost because improvement comes quickly and is easily measured. "You might start off lifting 20 pounds, but soon you have to put more weight on the bar or lower the pin to a different position," he says. You don't need huge muscle gains to reap the benefits—all you need is enough so you perceive that something has changed. That happens readily with lifting because you're expecting to see change, says Dr. Tucker.

Good feelings about your body can spill positive feelings into other parts of life, too, says Dr. Tucker. "An awful lot of the confidence in everything we do stems from how we perceive our bodies," he says. Your barbells may be a good way to shatter the bad body image that's keeping you back.

ten seconds. Relax, then bend your fingers in at the knuckles and hold for ten seconds. Repeat.

Shoulder shrug. For shoulders, upper and middle back. Raise your shoulders toward your ears until you feel a slight tension in your neck and shoulders. Hold five seconds, then relax your shoulders downward into their normal position. Repeat two or three times.

Arm extension. For shoulders, middle and upper back, sides, arms, hands and fingers. Interlace your fingers, palms facing out, and straighten your arms, at shoulderheight, in front of you. Feel a stretch through your arms and shoulder blades. Hold for 20 to 30 seconds. Then, bring your straightened arms overhead, elongating your spine as you feel a stretch through your arms and the upper sides of your rib cage. Hold 20 to 30 seconds. Repeat two times.

Standing

Back extension. For lower back and chest. Bend your knees slightly and place your palms on your lower back just above your hips, fingers pointing downward. Gently push your palms into your lower back; hold comfortable pressure for 10 to 15 seconds. Repeat two times. Use this stretch after sitting for an extended period of time.

Trunk twist. For spine, lower back and hips. With your hands on your hips, knees slightly bent and toes pointed forward, rotate your hips to the right as you look over your right shoulder behind you. Hold an easy stretch for 10 to 15 seconds. Repeat two times on each side.

Neck pull. To stretch the side of your neck and top of your shoulder, lean your head sideways toward your left shoulder as your left hand pulls your right arm down and across behind your back. Hold an easy stretch for ten seconds. Do both sides. This stretch can be done sitting on the floor, in a chair or while standing.

A Rundown of the Top Flab-Fighting Exercises

We like to know what we stand to gain from our efforts. In the case of aerobic exercise, we like to know what we stand to lose. Call it incentive. So the following chart shows you exactly how many pounds you can expect to drop by getting some regular exercise. Just 40 minutes of one of the following activities three days a week will leave you lighter and trimmer in less than two months. Want to lose even more weight? Start watching what you're eating more closely. By trimming just 250 calories from your daily diet, the amount in 2½ tablespoons of butter, you'll lose an additional four pounds in the same time.

Activity	Calories burned in 40 min.	Total weight lost after 8 weeks at 3×/week (lb.)
Basketball	472	3.2
Boxing (sparring)	440	3.0
Cycling (9.4 mph)	320	2.2
Frisbee	320	2.2
Golf	272	1.9
Jogging (7 min./mile)	716	4.9
Jumping rope (80/min.)	524	3.6
Scuba diving	568	3.9
Softball	220	1.5
Stair-climbing	540	3.7
Swimming (slow crawl)	408	2.8
Tennis	460	3.2
Volleyball	472	3.2
Walking (4 mph)	312	2.1

* Figures based on a 176-pound man

Calf stretch. For calf muscles. Stand at least two feet from a wall. Cross your forearms and lean them on the wall, resting your head on your arms. With your right foot in front, knee bent, extend your straightened left leg behind, heel to ground and toes forward. Slowly move your hips forward until you feel a stretch in your calf. Hold for 15 to 20 seconds. Repeat with your right leg.

Quadriceps stretch. For the front of the thigh. Holding on to support with your left hand, grasp the top of your left foot behind you with your right hand. Gently pull your heel toward your buttocks. Hold 15 to 20 seconds. Repeat for your right leg.

Source: This chapter was excerpted from *Computer and Desk Stretches* by Bob and Jean Anderson of Stretching Inc.

Part Seven

Striding to Slimness

Walk This Way

You've probably picked up a few bad habits since you were four years old. Here are ten steps to get you back on track.

An evolutionary imperative sings in our infant blood. "Come on, baby—do the locomotion," it croons. Baby needs little coaxing.

"Nobody teaches us how to walk," says James Gage, an orthopedist at the University of Minnesota. "We just do it, when we're about a year old. Our gait develops until the age of 3½ to 4, and then we're walking in an adult pattern, similar to anybody else's."

Then why are folks trying to make the primal act of peregrination seem so difficult? Perhaps because there's money in knocking our walking. Take one magazine article declaring that previously undetected toe defects are tripping up nearly 110 percent of the population. The one thing that would save strolling as we know it? An expensive corrective device that is available only from the practitioner who issued the urgent diagnosis and wrote the story.

Then there was the physician who contacted a fitness research center hoping for an endorsement. He'd acquire financial backing for his discovery of a whole new way to walk. "But all he'd done," says the expert who reviewed his work, "was break down the components of traditional race walking and rename it the Dr. So-and-So Walking Technique, to be promoted in an expensive book." Just as pricey but downright dangerous, says the reviewer, was another product sent for official approval—a belt with rubber bands that you're supposed to push and pull while you walk, as if you're a living Nautilus machine. "We tried it," says the reviewer, "and we found out the belt tightens as you pull, making it hard to breathe. But it's on the market!"

Is the act of ambulation really so esoteric that it requires special devices and new names—pace walking, space walking, cake walking and Dr. So-and-So walking? Would we really risk injury and humiliation if we engaged in just plain walking, holding the modifiers? At what point should this matter be referred the Ministry of Silly Walks? We decided to ask the experts.

"The walker's motto should be 'Keep it simple and do what comes naturally,' " says cardiologist James Rippe, M.D., director of the exercise physiology and nutrition laboratory at the University of Massachusetts Medical School in Worcester and co-author of *Fitness Walking for Women.* "For most people, the right way to walk is more or less what they're already doing. If you're asked to learn something terribly complex, chances are it's not worth learning."

"People know how to walk," says Gage. "We just need to train them in endurance, to correct bad posture, which leads to chronic back problems, and to make a few other minor adjustments."

Natural-born walkers lapse into less-than-perfect tendencies over the course of a lifetime. In these pages, our experts review the moves you once made intuitively—and will make again.

A Walker's Ten Commandments

1. Your head is high. Not too high; the underside of your chin should be parallel to the ground. "It's a small change that makes a big difference," says Joseph Askinasi, a New York City kinesiologist and chiropractor. "I sympathize with urban walkers trying not to put their foot in it, but tilting your head down prevents efficient breathing, changes the curve of your spine, strains the neck, shoulders and back and increases fatigue."

2. Your stomach is pulled in. Do what you'd do reflexively if someone ordered you to suck in your gut; you'll feel a tightening of the stomach and a lifting of the chest. If you walk with a loose belly, you risk painful back strain, says Ellen Abbott, a fitness consultant in Brookline, Massachusetts. "In general, poor posture makes you tire faster and contributes to join and muscle soreness."

Let's cross-check before taking off. At the beginning (and middle and end) of every walk, you're standing tall, with your shoulders pulled back and relaxed and your chest leading you. (A sunken chest is no treasure; you can't breathe efficiently.) Your abdominal muscles are pulled in and up, and your gluteals—butt muscles—are pulled forward under the hips, causing the slightest of pelvic tilts.

3. Your arms swing in moderation. "No rocking-the-baby or windshield-wiper arms," says Wendy Oakes, associate director of the Cooper Fitness Center of the Cooper Aerobics Center in Dallas. "Your arms should swing in natural opposition to your feet." Starting at the hip, each elbow should move forward along an arc finishing no higher than your breastbone, then return for an equal arc backward. Don't swivel your hips, Oakes says, and don't shake your booty.

4. You find your natural stride. "A lot of people take giant steps thinking that they're improving efficiency," says Oakes, "when they're actually inhibiting it." Steps that are too long overwork the calf muscle responsible for breaking the propulsion forward. Also avoid locking your knee in a hyperextended position.

Oakes says most people can find a comfortable stride. Or try this test: Stand with feet slightly apart and parallel, heels on the ground, then lean forward until you have to take a step to keep from falling over. "That's your natural stride," says Oakes.

5. You step lightly. No galumphing. "You should be walking heel-ball-toe," says Abbott. "Land on your heel, flex your toes toward the sky, roll through the foot and finally push off. Walking is rocking—it's the rock that perpetuates the forward roll."

Good posture creates lightness of step, says Askinasi. Imagine a string pulling you up from the top of your head. "You shouldn't be able to hear your feet. You don't have to walk around like a ninja, but that heavy boom-bada-boom shouldn't be there. I urge people to go for a while without a Walkman, to make sure their feet aren't making noise."

6. You stop and stretch. "Start off walking slowly for five to ten minutes, then stretch," says Abbott. "Warmed-up muscles stretch more efficiently and safely." Stretching pays off in speed and grace and prevents soreness and injury.

It's especially crucial after cooldown. "Your muscles burn glucose and fat to produce energy, creating an 'exhaust' of mostly lactic acid," says Askinasi. "If you go home and sit, the lactic acid in your muscles will cause them to tighten. Stretching helps to pump the acid out. The more fit you are,

A Word to the Inert . . .

Would the rest of you give us some privacy?

Yo! You on the chaise eating bonbons (and when I say you, I mean me). You poised on the corner of walk and don't walk. No more excuses. You now have everything to gain from joining the movement.

First: Even nonaerobic exercise earns you big health benefits. "For a long time, we confused aerobic fitness—working within the heart-rate target zone—with health. And that may be why such a high percentage of Americans do not exercise," says Lorna Francis, professor of physical education at San Diego State University. "The thought of having to reach your target zone for 20 minutes three to five times a week was daunting." But some studies have found that moderate exercise for 20 or 30 minutes every day or so, while not doing much for cardiovascular fitness, still greatly lowers risk for heart disease, stroke, diabetes, osteoporosis and prostate, colon and breast cancers.

Second: You can accumulate that walking time during a day. "We made a mistake in thinking the activity has to occur all in one session," says Steven Blair, P.E.D., director of epidemiology at the Cooper Institute for Aerobics Research in Dallas. "If you're typing all day, and you take a 2-minute walk every two hours, the general notion is you're likely to get benefits comparable to those from a 16-minute walk."

In other words, it's better to do little bits of activity—such as getting off the bus a stop early and walking and climbing stairs instead of taking the elevator—than one big hunk of nothing. "The five-mile run you don't take isn't going to do you a bit of good," says Dr. Blair, "while the three ten-minute walks you might manage to fit in will do you more good than sitting."

. . . And to the Highly "Ert"

If you're after more than fabulous health benefits, if you want optimum cardiovascular fitness, prepare to enter the target zone. Here's how to know you've made it.

- Calculate your maximum heart rate per minute—how fast your ticker is likely to tock during aerobic activity—by subtracting your age from 220.
- Your target zone to get aerobic fitness is any heart rate between 60 and 90 percent of this maximum. Multiply the maximum by 0.6 and then by 0.9 to find the zone's bottom and top.
- During a workout, stop and take your pulse for 15 seconds, then multiply by four. That's your per-minute heart rate. Is it within your target zone?
- Take your pulse at different times—the beginning of your walk, at top stride, during cooldown—during several different walks. Try guessing your heart rate, then confirm it with a count. Studies show that walkers can eventually tell whether their heart rates are in the target zone without taking their pulses.
- You'll know you're pushing too hard if you're too winded to walk and carry on a conversation at the same time.

the faster you naturally clear out the exhaust. But even fit people have to stretch."

Do this simple stretch even on days you don't walk, suggests sports podiatrist Stephen Pribut of Washington, D.C. Use your arms to lean against a wall, as if you were pushing it, and place one foot a stride forward with the knee bent. Keeping both heels on the ground, ease into the wall until you feel the stretch in the calf of the back leg. Stretch each leg for ten seconds up to ten times until loose.

7. You know your limits. "The person who begins a walking a program, walks for 20 minutes, then says 'I feel great! I'll do an hour!' won't feel great the next morning," says Askinasi. If you're not in shape, keep your workout to 20 minutes a day for a least two weeks. Otherwise you'll be much more likely to begin suffering from interior tibialis pain, a soreness often confused with shin splints, which comes from stretching or tearing the muscle where it attaches to the shin bone. "The tibialis is easily fatigued and hard to stretch out," says Oakes. "Warm it up thoroughly." She suggests that you get blood flowing to the muscle by standing and steadying yourself against a wall or fence and rotating the foot slowly in the air. Do that ten times clockwise and ten times counterclockwise, then repeat with the other foot.

8. You travel empty-handed. No hand weights. "People perceive they're working harder when they're holding two-pound weights," says Abbott, "but they're not burning any more calories, and they're putting undue strain on joints and muscles, especially those of the hand and forearm."

Adds Dr. Rippe, "The right arm counterbalances the left leg and vice versa. Weight one or the other, and you throw off a very delicate balance, increasing the risk of injury to elbows and shoulders and to delicate leg structures, particularly the knees."

If you want to work harder, increase your speed or change terrain. Go uphill, walk on sand or into the wind. (You'll get a zephyr-assisted return trip.) If you want to build your upper body, weight-training is fine—but not while you're walking.

Of course, if you often walk to work or around town while carrying a purse or briefcase, you can't use the no-hand-weights rule as an excuse to jump in a cab. Empty hands are ideal, but walking with a handful is better than not walking at all.

9. You drink your fill. Dehydration can lead to a weak stride, light-headedness, headache, sore muscles, unsightly facial hair, horrid age spots and waxy yellow buildup. All right, we lied about the last three. But you should be drinking eight eight-ounce glasses of water a day. The beverage police have their eyes on you.

10. You know that walking isn't wimpy. To some folks, walking doesn't seem difficult enough. "How can I possibly be extending my life," they say, aghast, "if I'm not killing myself?"

They can rest easy (or rest hard, if they prefer), says Dr. Rippe. Most people—85 percent of the 1,000 that Dr. Rippe followed in one study—can start getting the benefits of an aerobic workout simply by picking up their pace a bit from three miles an hour, which is the average speed at which we move through the daily business of life. "Walking at four miles an hour requires no different biomechanical motions than everyday walking," says Dr. Rippe. "And yet you get into the target heart zone. When you want to further improve your aerobic fitness, you can accelerate to five miles per hour.

"If you think that's not vigorous—four laps of a standard track in 12 minutes—try it and find out how brisk walking can be," he says. Even a group of young marathoners that Dr. Rippe studies were able to hit their target training zones walking—at five miles an hour. That's as fast as you can walk without getting a coach and taking up technical race walking.

(continued on page 194)

How to Choose Your Shoes

The risk of serious injury is low for walkers. One study found that even race walkers sustain significant injuries, such as a sprained ankle or torn ligament, only once every 51.7 years. The walking wounded are more likely to suffer chronic strains or soreness. Stretching and heeding pain early will help you avoid these. So will wearing good shoes. But how do we know what's good? We're wooed by Bo, Michael and Paula, each offering irresistible shoes equipped with gel, a dial, a pump, a wet bar, a sunken tub and a changing room. Must we get so fancy? Here's what counts.

Stick to walking shoes. Though it's not a sin to walk in a running shoe, most of them have a more flexible sole and a higher heel than a regular fitness walker wants.

Go for instant comfort. Walking shoes should feel right as soon as you put them on without the temporary pinch and bind you might tolerate in dress shoes.

Shop at the time of day you walk. Remember that as blood pools during the day—the price of walking upright— your feet get bigger by up to three-quarters of a shoe size. So try on shoes when you normally walk—and wear your usual walking socks.

Try on both shoes. Many of us have one foot that's longer than the other. Concentrate on whether the shoe fits the longer foot.

Search your sole. "Shoe flexibility at the ball of the foot is very important," says sports podiatrist Stephen Pribut of Washington, D.C. "That's the only place where the shoe should bend. If it isn't stable up to that point, you could be liable to twisting and turning, and your arch is vulnerable. Flex the shoe to make sure. You've just done 80 percent of the work of successful shoe shopping."

Go for a snug heel. Your heel should be hugged by the shoe. "The hard piece that fits around the back of the shoe— the heel counter—should be firm," says Pribut. "It should continue at least 20 percent of the length of the shoe toward the toe on either side. You can gauge its firmness by squeezing it." If the counter cups the heel without sliding up and down, that will help prevent pronation, a turning in of the foot that forces the arch to lower.

Search the store. In general, women have a higher arch and a narrower heel than men, but this isn't true for all women. "If a woman has a large, wide foot," Pribut says, "she shouldn't feel funny about wearing a man's shoe."

Check the cushioning. If you think you're too lightweight to need a lot of cushioning, consider that up to $1^1/_2$ times your body weight goes through the heel on each foot strike. If that shock isn't dispersed by the shoe, it'll be absorbed by ankles, knees and hips. Generally, the higher your arch, the more cushioning you need.

Wear dry, padded socks. Polypropylene wicks moisture away from the foot. Many walkers say a blend of polypropylene and wool or cotton is even more comfortable. Padded socks fight blisters and promote bliss.

Don't forget they're new shoes. "The biggest error made by even experienced walkers is wearing new shoes and going for a longer walk than usual," says Pribut. The result is blisters, ankle soreness and other nagging injuries. The newly shod should trim their walk by 20 percent for three or four days, Pribut recommends, no matter how comfortable the shoes.

Buy a new pair every 400 hours of walking. If it were only the shoe companies sounding this warning, we might be suspicious, but who can ignore a pair of barking dogs? If your shoes are worn out, Pribut says, you're at risk of forefoot soreness and even a stress fracture, one of those rare serious walking wounds.

"I don't tell patients what brand to use," he says. "I send them to a reputable athletic-shoe store or suggest that they call a walking group or running club and ask where their members go to get a good fit."

The dedicated brisk walker accrues the same aerobic fitness as a runner, but with a lower risk of injury, Dr. Rippe says; a runner hits the ground with a force 3 to 4 times the body's weight, while a walker hits with only 1 to 1½ times.

How do you know when you've broken the brisk barrier? One way is to time yourself on a track. "But Harry Truman defined it better than anyone," Dr. Rippe says. "A Secret Service man escorting the president asked what pace he should set. President Truman answered, 'Walk as though you have someplace to go.'"

—*Judith Stone*

Unwind with a Mindful Stroll

Use meditation techniques to multiply your walk's positive mental benefits.

We know that aerobic exercise has the power to calm jangled nerves and boost drooping moods. Research has shown that one brisk 20- to 30-minute walk can have the same calming effect as a mild tranquilizer. And we know that over time, a regular exercise program can enhance self-esteem and reduce depression. But now there's research suggesting that even something less vigorous than a brisk walk—a comfortable stroll—can leave you feeling less anxious and more positive. By adding simple mental techniques, strollers get the same positive mental benefits that brisk walkers enjoy.

The Body/Mind Connection

Researchers from three institutions brought together their expertise to see how "cognitive," or "mindful," exercises might enhance the effect of exercise on the body and mind. The study was conducted by Ruth Stricker, owner and director of The Marsh: A Center for Balance and Fitness in Minnetonka, Minnesota, and James Rippe, M.D., director of the exercise physiology and nutrition laboratory at the University of Massachusetts Medical School in Worcester.

This research, called the Ruth Stricker/MindBody Study, investigated five groups (135 people in all) over a 16-week period. Of the three walking groups, one walked at a brisk pace, one at a low-intensity pace and one at a low-intensity pace with an extra element.

This latter group practiced a mental technique to bring about the "relaxation response" developed by Herbert Benson, M.D., president of New England Deaconess Hospital's Mind/Body Medical Institute in Boston, in an attempt to see how the mind and body work together. This relaxation response is a physiological response characterized by decreased heart rate and blood pressure and feelings of tranquillity. The fourth group practiced mindful exercise—a Westernized application of tai chi developed by Stricker. The fifth group served as controls and were asked not to change anything about their lives.

The low-intensity walkers using the mental technique listened to a tape that explained that while exercise and relaxation techniques seem very different, they actually produce very similar results through the power of repetition. They were instructed in how to do a simple meditation. They were asked to pay attention to their footsteps during their walks, counting one, two, one, two. They were also instructed to visualize the numbers in their minds. If they found their thoughts drifting, they were to say "Oh, well" and come back to counting their footsteps.

The results of using this simple technique were "dramatic," according to Dr. Rippe. The low-intensity walking group that used the relaxation tape showed decreases in anxiety and had fewer negative and more positive feelings about themselves—equal to the effect that the brisk walkers gained. These effects were evident after just one exercise session and were maintained over the duration of the study. The low-intensity walkers who did not use the mental technique showed no improvements until the 14th week, but even the improvements were not as extensive. The group that practiced mindful exercise experienced very similar results to the group that used the mental technique, lending support to the idea that various cognitive strategies can yield similar benefits.

"For people who have difficulty with brisk walking or other moderately intense exercise, this is a very encouraging study," says Dr. Rippe. "They can be encouraged to exercise knowing that with a simple mental technique, they can get the same psychological benefits as a person who can exercise at a higher intensity."

This type of research may prove even more fruitful in the future, says David Brown, Ph.D., research psychologist at the Centers for Disease Control and Prevention in Atlanta, who designed the study. "In the Ruth Stricker/MindBody Study, we used healthy volunteers from the general population. They did not have any physical disabilities, nor were they abnormally anxious or depressed. It's difficult to get improved ratings on psychological tests when your subject already feels just fine. I believe a study done with a clinical population, a group of people experiencing physical limitations or mental distress, would show even greater improvement from the walking/mindful approach."

Exercise Inspiration

Many people know that exercise is beneficial. In fact, a survey showed 93 percent of adults think that exercise is good for them. Yet only 20 percent of Americans exercise regularly.

"It's certainly not that they don't have enough information," says Dr. Rippe. "But maybe it's a bit overwhelming to some people to think they have to maintain their exercise for weeks, even years, to gain those health benefits. This study shows people that they can experience almost immediate psychological benefits, that they can feel better from exercise right away, even if they can't move at a fast pace. Maybe when people are educated about exercise in this way, they'll be more inclined to give it a try and more likely to stay with it."

Deena and David Balboa, co-directors of the Walking Center of New York City, think this study confirms what they've experienced for years in working with hundreds of clients. "We teach people to tune in to their bodies when they walk," the Balboas explain. "It doesn't matter what mindful technique you use. If you concentrate on your body, whether it's your form, rhythm, posture or breathing, a calming takes effect as body awareness increases. Just moving in an unconscious fashion can't produce the harmony and aliveness that emerge naturally from being mindful during exercise."

—Maggie Spilner

Pair Up and Do Double Time

Find a walking buddy or two and improve your stick-to-it power.

Although people can undertake many exercise programs by themselves, studies have shown that very few of them start or continue unless they have partners. People need social support. Even when people join groups, they generally do it along with friends.

Walking seems special in that many of us love the time we spend during solitary walks. But most of us find that having partners keeps us going when our motivation starts to slide and we think we have too many other "more important" things to do.

Wise Choices for Walkers

If you want to reap the physical and mental benefits of walking, it should become an almost daily activity for the rest of your life. So when you go searching for a partner, it seems like a good idea to stay close to home. See if you can enlist your spouse, child, parent, close neighbor or even family dog. That way, each time you exercise, you also strengthen the relationships that are most important in your life, those that help maintain your sense of happiness and well-being.

Some days you choose your walking partners, and some days they choose you. Be open and flexible to whoever happens to walk your way! You may not find someone who shares your enthusiasm for walking every day, but you may find two or three different people to keep you company throughout the week.

Pairing Up with a Pooch

It's not for everyone, and we would never recommend buying a pet just to have a walking partner. But hundreds of letters from *Prevention* magazine's Walking Club members over the years have convinced us that a dog can be a most reliable walking buddy.

Dogs always want to go for walks and tend to be very enthusiastic about the whole idea. They remind you when it is time to go (in case you've forgotten or gotten too comfortable in front of the TV). And they make good company. They rarely complain and are great listeners if you want to talk. And if you decide to wear headphones and listen to music or a good book, a dog won't feel slighted.

Dogs may need some sort of obedience training to make your partnership enjoyable, but most are able walking partners right from the start. If you don't already have a dog, check with a local veterinarian or kennel club as to which breed would best suit your needs and your family's lifestyle.

If you have a dog who has not been exercised regularly, let your vet examine him and then advise you how far and how fast he can go as he warms up to your walking program.

The Kid Connection

Children can be great walking partners, provided you're walking toward some destination they have a great interest in. If you ask your son or daughter to just "go for a walk," there's a good chance you will be either ignored or ridiculed. But kids love to walk to video arcades, ice-cream parlors or baseball-card stores. The distance never seems to be daunting if the end goal is enticing enough. And you can have lots of fun and exercise along the way.

When walking with young kids, remember: You're the adult, the one with the ability to adapt. Walk slowly enough to match their pace. Don't walk so far or so fast that they'll never trust you enough to go with you again. And don't take it as an opportunity to lecture to a captive audience. Smile. Relax. Let them talk, and enjoy their company.

Walking at Work

The workplace can be fertile ground for finding walking partners. Everybody gets breaks, and a walk break can be a better stress reducer and rejuvenator than coffee or a doughnut.

Try to plan at least some of your lunch hour as walking time, too. Don't skip your meal, but even a 15-minute walk is a great stress reliever.

Look for different partners for different kinds of walking. On days you're not up to working up a sweat, find somebody who likes to stroll. Find someone else for those ½-hour hill strides that are worth 1½ hours of level walking. Walking with people you work with allows you to get to know each other outside the pressures of the job. You may develop an easygoing rapport along with a better-toned body!

Keep an extra pair of walking shoes and socks at work

so you can be ready at a moment's notice. For really brisk walking on a warm day, you may want to change into athletic clothing. But on cool days, just slipping into your comfy walking shoes can energize you for a brisk walk.

Try to find partners who are generally equal to you in stamina. Don't try to keep up with anyone who is really too fast for you. It's not worth the risk of injury. If they are carrying on most of the conversation as you gasp for breath, slow down!

Walking on Common Ground

To keep motivation high, it's best if your most frequent walking partners have the same agenda as you. They want to lose weight, work off stress, increase their endurance and general fitness level or all of the above. Maybe you both like to bird-watch or enjoy window shopping while you walk. Whatever pleasures or goals you have in common will help to bring you together again and again for health-building walks.

—Maggie Spilner

Hit the Great Indoors
for Winter Workouts

When the north wind blows, try these cozy alternatives.

For many people, winter is a favorite time for brisk walks. When you're dressed in properly layered clothing, the cold air can be invigorating and refreshing.

But for some of us, winter weather is a problem—either because icy, snowy conditions make walking hazardous or because we have health factors that make cold weather too stressful to be safe.

"Talk to your doctor if you have heart disease or diabetes," says specialist in aging and exercise William M. Simpson Jr., M.D., professor of family medicine at the Medical University of South Carolina in Charleston. "Many people with heart disease can gradually acclimate to cold weather. As long as you walk almost daily, your body will cope with the demands of cold weather."

Since cold weather does stress the body (burning more calories), people with diabetes may experience trouble with low blood sugar when they exercise outdoors. They may need to acclimate gradually or adjust their insulin. And they need to be very careful about their hands and feet if they have difficulty feeling temperature. Double socks in shoes large enough to accommodate them can help. Warm gloves or mittens are a must.

"People with arthritis need to allow more time for their joints to warm up," says Dr. Simpson. "And people with asthma may find it necessary to pretreat themselves with bronchodilator medication and/or wear a mask to help warm the air they breathe."

If a particularly bad cold spell is temporary, say just a few weeks, don't worry that you'll lose all your fitness benefits overnight.

"In general, cardiovascular fitness is lost at half the rate at which it was attained," says Wayne Westcott, Ph.D., *Prevention* magazine advisor and strength consultant to the YMCA and the National Academy of Sports Medicine.

"For example," he says, "if you're healthy and you build up your fitness level by walking for 10 weeks and then you stop, but not because of injury or sickness, it would take about 20 weeks to lose the fitness you gained in that 10 weeks."

Moving Indoors

If health factors or freezing temperatures force you indoors for a whole season, you'll need indoor alternatives to maintain your fitness level. The least-expensive indoor alternative is mall walking.

According to Tom Cabot, president of the National Organization of Mall Walkers, there are over 3,000 enclosed malls in the United States, and about 80 percent of them have walking programs.

Dorothy Winfield and Mary Ann Trempt of Kenosha, Wisconsin, have been walking year-round in the Factory Outlet Mall since 1987. "We enjoy the walking, and we really look forward to being with the group that has formed," says Winfield. Once around the inside of the mall is nine-tenths of a mile, and walkers show up beginning at 7:00 A.M., when the doors open just for them. Many walk four miles or more. Their group socializes in the mall after walking, and they plan additional activities like bus trips, card parties and holiday parties. "We even keep a picture album of our different activities," Winfield says.

Muscle-Specific Machines

"Walking involves lifting your center of gravity with every step," says Dr. Westcott. "You're moving vertically and horizontally. In order to keep those same muscles active and fit, the most similar indoor activity would be walking on a treadmill."

Treadmills are available at health clubs. If you want to buy a quality treadmill to use at home, you'll need to spend at least $600.

"The next-best type of exercise equipment for a walker's indoor workout would be a stair-climbing machine," says Dr. Westcott. "You use the same muscles that you would use walking uphill." Again, stair-climbing machines are available in most health clubs. Home models can cost from $200 for a mechanical type to $3,000 for a computerized version. (You could climb the stairs at home, but coming back down puts too much stress on joints and muscles.)

A less-expensive alternative to stair-climbers, but which uses the same muscles, is bench-stepping. Benches cost from $50 to $100. You can exercise to a video at home or join a class at the local YMCA, where benches are provided.

"Cross-country ski machines are the next closest exercise," says Dr. Westcott. "You lose the vertical component because you never lift your feet off the ground, but you have extended horizontal movement. And using the arms stresses the cardiovascular system more, which, in a way, compensates for the lack of vertical work." Quality cross-country ski machines can be purchased for around $400.

Many people wonder how a stationary bike compares with walking for exercise. "Bicycles and rowing machines use many of the same leg muscles that walking does, but in a different way. Your weight is supported, so there is no pull against gravity," says Dr. Westcott. "But you can get a great cardiovascular workout on a stationary bike, and in the spring, when you start walking outdoors again, you'd get in shape very quickly, since you wouldn't have lost your general cardiovascular fitness level." You'd have the energy to walk; you'd just need a few days or weeks to get certain muscles used to walking again. And you might experience a little muscle soreness. Exercise bikes range in price from $200 for a quality bike to $2,000 for a high-tech version.

Remember, prices for most of the fitness equipment available vary depending on your fitness goals and the features of each machine.

—Maggie Spilner

Part Eight
Stay Psyched

Homework

No time to make it to the gym? Sneak in a sweat at home with this simple low-tech, high-gain fitness routine.

> *'Mid pleasures and palaces though we may roam, Be it ever so humble, there's no place like home.*

John Howard Payne may not have had a penchant for exercise, but his rhyme certainly applies to people who do—although few may realize it. "Most people think they can exercise only if they belong to a gym," says Stacy Fowler, a personal trainer in Beverly Hills, California, whose clients refer to her as Proud Coach. "But that's a ridiculous excuse. In fact, with a little creativity, any home can serve as a perfectly adequate gym."

As the proud owner of a state-of-the-art home gym for which she paid $20,000, Fowler puts her money where her mouth is. But don't worry, she says; you don't have to blow a wad to construct yours. In fact, you're not likely to need any new supplies whatsoever.

"You can fill plastic bottles with water or sand and use them as dumbbells," she says. "A bathroom shower stall is all you need for stretches and flexibility exercises. And a broom can help you perform easy torso twists and squats." Need an aerobic challenge? Climb stairs or head out the front door for a brisk walk. That's how Fowler shed 59 pounds after giving birth to her first child, Presley Ann, last year.

A No-Excuses Exercise Plan

Ready to give the no-tech approach a whirl? We'll provide your first nudge with Fowler's room-by-room guide to home-based fitness. Her unapologetically simple plan requires only three things in the way of "equipment"—a house or apartment, some props from the hall or kitchen closet and just a touch of down-home motivation and stick-to-itiveness.

"There isn't a single person who shouldn't be able to make time for this," says Fowler. "So don't make excuses. Simply follow the plan, and 'sneak' exercise into your daily life." Begin by performing the routine two or three times per week, then increase your frequency to five times a week as your strength and fitness improve.

First things first: When you go to bed tonight, set your alarm to sound five or ten minutes earlier than usual. Proud Coach's home fitness program starts as soon as your day starts—in the bedroom.

Bedroom Biz

You needn't get out of the sack to begin. Simply lie on your back with your head flat on the mattress, and pull your knees to your chest. Hold for 30 seconds, then return to the starting position. Repeat, this time bringing your bent legs to your right and left sides, again keeping your shoulders and upper back flat on the bed. Then get out of bed, and repeat the sequence while lying on the floor, which will offer greater support for your lower back—the area you're targeting with this morning stretch.

Next, you'll address your abdominals. Remain on your back on the floor with your knees bent. Place your heels flat on the floor, shoulder-width apart and as close to your buttocks as comfortably possible. Resist hooking your feet under the edge of the bed; this allows you to use your legs during the exercise, and you want to isolate your abs. Fold your hands over your abdomen; keep your elbows relaxed and out to the side and your chin away from your chest.

Gradually curl up, lifting your head and shoulders by contracting your abs; exhale for a count of five as you go. Pause when your lower back is pressed flat into the floor. Inhale, and lower your torso, again counting to five until your shoulder blades touch the floor. Try not to relax your abs before you begin your next crunch. You should feel the burn in the muscles above your belly button. Begin with five to ten crunches per session, adding more as your strength improves. Next, hit the shower.

Bathroom Stretch

Singing isn't the only sort of performing you can do in the shower—you can stretch your calves and quadriceps (thighs) there, too. The combination of moist heat and the following movements works wonders.

To stretch your quads, steady yourself by placing your left hand against the wall or shower stall, then grab your right ankle with your right hand as you lift your right foot directly backward toward your buttocks. Hold for 30 seconds, then repeat the stretch with your other leg.

Next, move to the back of the shower for two calf stretches; use a bath mat if the floor of your shower is slippery. To stretch the calf muscle called the gastrocnemius, stand facing the wall of the shower, about an arm's length away. Place both palms flat against the wall and lean in by bending your elbows, keeping your body straight and your heels flat on the floor. Hold for 30 seconds, then relax and repeat five times. To stretch the soleus (your other calf muscle), assume the same position as you did to stretch the gastrocnemius, but bend your knees slightly as you lean into the wall. Hold for 30 seconds, then relax and repeat five times.

Kitchen Contortions

If you struggle to make it to work on time every day, you may want to hold off on these exercises until dinnertime. But if your schedule permits, Fowler suggests trying them while the bagels brown and the coffee percolates.

To start, use your kitchen countertop as a ballet bar. Stand a few feet away, facing the counter with your feet pointing forward. Then lift one leg and rest it on the counter (or wrap your toes around the counter's edge). Keeping your leg straight, gradually lean your upper body forward, toward your foot, stretching out your arms as if to touch your toes. Hold for 20 to 30 seconds. Do not bounce. Feel the tightness in your hamstrings (the muscles stretching from the back of your knee up to your buttocks). Then repeat with your other leg.

Next, grab a broom and rest it on top of your shoulders (behind your head and neck). Grasp the broom handle with both hands, and twist slowly from side to side, using the broom to keep your body within a single plane. Twist for 10 to 20 repetitions or until your torso and arms feel the stretch.

Now that you're warmed up, you're ready to squat to strengthen your hamstrings and buttocks. With the broom still on your shoulders, stand with your feet parallel and roughly shoulder-width apart. Grasp the broom handle with both hands, about shoulder-width apart. With your head up and back straight, squat until your upper thighs are almost parallel to the floor. (Your buttocks should not drop below knee level.) If this is uncomfortable, squat as far as you can, then return to the starting position. Take five to ten seconds each on the descent and ascent. Start with 5 squats, and gradually progress to 20 as your strength improves.

Family-Room Fun

Can't give up your "Jeopardy"? Then lift weights while you watch. To fashion your own dumbbells, simply fill two medium-size water bottles with tap water, sand or dirt, and weigh them on your bathroom scale to see how much you'll be lifting. Depending on their size, the bottles may weigh from 2 to 15 pounds each.

Start with two-pounders, and try some lateral raises to strengthen your deltoids (shoulder muscles): Stand erect with a bottle in each hand and your arms at your sides. Then slowly raise your arms straight outward to shoulder level, hold for an instant and return to the starting position. Repeat 10 to 15 times, increasing the weight as your strength improves.

Next, try a few lunges: Stand erect with a two-pound bottle in each hand, your arms at your sides and your feet parallel and about shoulder-width apart. Leading with your right leg, lunge forward as far as possible, gently bending your knee over your toes until your right thigh is almost parallel to the floor; don't allow your knee to extend past your toes. Your left knee should bend down toward the floor. Push back to the starting position, and repeat 10 to 20 times. Then repeat with your left leg. Increase the weight as your strength improves.

A word of caution: Lunges can stress the front surface of your knee if they're performed improperly. If you feel pain in your knee as you lunge, stop immediately.

Excess Doesn't Spell Success

Think you can never be too rich, too thin—or too aerobicized? Think again. Just as you can diet too much, you can exercise too much. And the results can be equally disastrous.

"The tricky part about addiction to exercise is that it sounds like it's good for you," says Jorge de la Torre, M.D., assistant professor of psychiatry at Baylor College of Medicine in Houston. "And this makes the problem difficult to identify. Yet in many ways, exercise addiction can be as damaging as an addiction to drugs or alcohol."

Just as substance abusers often neglect areas of their lives not associated with their addiction, obsessive exercisers consume themselves with lengthy workouts, often to the detriment of their health, marriage, job performance and family life.

If you fear that you're overdoing it, try to shorten your daily exercise sessions in nonthreatening increments. You might start by trimming one minute per session each week if that's all you can manage to give up. From there, gradually shoot for resting completely at least one day a week. If these changes make you anxious or depressed, or if you resume your old routine in short order, consult your doctor for a referral to a therapist.

On to bicep (upper arm) curls: Stand erect with your feet shoulder-width apart and your knees slightly bent. Grasp a two-pound bottle in each hand, with your arms at your sides. Bend your elbows to lift the bottles slowly with your palms facing upward. Stop just before your elbows form 90-degree angles. Repeat 10 to 15 times, increasing the weight as your strength improves.

Finally, try the bench press to build strength in your pectoral (chest) muscles: Lie on the floor on your back with your knees bent. Holding a two-pound bottle in each hand, bend your elbows at 90-degree angles and hold your arms perpendicular to your body. Slowly lift both bottles toward the ceiling at the same time, straightening your elbows as you lift. Pause at the top, then lower slowly. Repeat 10 to 15 times, increasing the weight as your strength improves.

There you have it—a results-guaranteed at-home fitness routine. Slim and shapely Dorothy had it right: There is no place like home—especially if you want to work out.

—Linda Miller

Five Hot New Ways to Stay Fit

The days of the go-for-the-burn workout are gone. The latest exercise trends are easy and playful and great for your health.

In the beginning, there was play. Then along came this thing called fitness. It was serious. It was intense. It required miles and miles of effort, crashing impact and a lot of guilt if you didn't "go for the burn." Problem was, all work and no play made fitness a dull sport. And many exercisers dropped out. But that was then. This is now. And the good news is that fitness in the 1990s is all about fun.

This doesn't mean that runners and aerobics fanatics have abandoned their sports. They've just begun to find ways to make them more fun. Road Runners Clubs across the country report soaring interest in team relays and other novelty events such as non-competitive fun runs. And aerobics studios are fast becoming indoor and outdoor playgrounds. For instance, Gin Miller, the instructor who made stepping up and down on a step bench a national aerobics pastime, has developed an adult exercise class that has participants running around obstacles, climbing up ropes and crawling through tunnels. She's now busy teaching her Step Reebok Circuit Challenge to instructors across the country. "The days of floor work with an instructor are over," says Miller. "There's a comfort zone in doing what we did as kids, and that's appealing."

Not to be outdone, Nike has come up with a class called Total Body Conditioning that uses a step bench, a slide, resistance bands and weights. Participants agree that it's a great workout, but what keeps them going back is that it's entertaining.

Of course, part of what's driving this new approach to staying in shape is that researchers have had time to evaluate the relative effect of high-intensity, strenuous workouts and less demanding activities on good health. Steven Blair, P.E.D., director of epidemiology at the Cooper Institute for Aerobics Research in Dallas, looked at the effects of exercise on mortality and found that moderate levels of activity were just as effective at prolonging life as high-intensity workouts, largely due to lower rates of heart disease and cancer. Moreover, it's now believed that 10-minute bouts of activity three times a day are as beneficial as one 30-minute workout. "Fitness in the 1980s became a rigid formula, another chore that you did with clenched teeth," says Ruth Stricker, owner and director of The Marsh: A Center for Balance and Fitness in Minnetonka, Minnesota. "We want to move beyond that and look at what is inherently good in exercise rather than what exercise is good for. We strive to replace failure and guilt with fun and joy."

That's what's happening in fitness. And even the scientists say it's a good idea. After all, when your workout is something you enjoy, you'll keep doing it, and it's not how hard you exercise that makes you healthier, it's how often. So if you're looking for a new workout, try one of these fun ways to stay fit.

The Outdoor Playground

Call it green fitness, if you like, but whatever the reason, environmental or otherwise, exercisers are moving outdoors—on mountain bikes, on foot, with ropes on cliffs. Fitness clubs are extending their boundaries through organized treks: ecology/hiking trips, kayaking weekends, in-line skate outings and backpacking adventures, for example. One indication of how popular this movement has become is the sales of outdoor gear. Nike reports a 29 percent increase in outdoor wear sales for this past summer. In addition, campsites are packed, and ski resorts are attracting climbers and bikers to their trails in the off-season.

A whole new crop of exercisers are getting off the beaten path and into the woods and spending their exercise time walking. Running clubs now offer walks with practically every road race. "A lot of people are out hiking, nature walking," says Bob Woodward, publisher of *SNEWS,* an outdoors-industry newsletter. In fact, the National Sporting Goods Association (NSGA) reports that hiking has increased in popularity by 24 percent from 1987 to 1992. Women, in particular, have taken up walking; 66 percent of the 67.8 million walkers in the United States are women.

Thomas Doyle, director of information and research at NSGA, predicts the trend will continue through the year 2000. How is he so sure? "First, those 45-plus-ers, the flower children of the 1970s, are raising families, and they have a kinship with the outdoors," says Doyle. "This dovetails very well with the so-called green movement in the United States and around the world."

Mergers and Marriages

The buzzword in aerobics is "cross-training." No more repetitive stepping. Now it's all-in-one classes that mix it up:

Exercise Reduces Potbellies Better

There's more than one way to lose a potbelly—but there's only one quick, surefire way. And that's exercise. In two studies of older men, those who dieted without exercising had to lose four times as much weight as exercisers in order to lose the same amount of abdominal fat!

Remember—not only is a potbelly a source of belt-expanding aggravation, it's also an obesity-related marker for heart disease, diabetes and high blood pressure. In this study, dieters needed to lose 20 pounds to skim off the same amount of fat from that region that exercisers trimmed by losing only 5 pounds. Somehow, the exercisers could more effectively target their weight loss.

Each study involved 20 volunteers. One group followed a strict 1,200-calorie-per-day limit for three months, while the other group continued their normal diets over the same period of time (in some cases increasing their food intakes) while exercising regularly.

"Exercise may be smarter in the long run than just dieting because it's a lot easier to keep off 5 pounds than it is to keep off 20," says Robert Schwartz, M.D., associate pro-

cardio-funk, high-low combo, step-sculpt, to name just a few. They'll work your heart, burn fat, improve your balance and agility and even get you to think about what your body is doing—all in a single, hour-long class. "The term *aerobics* has almost been thrown out," says Miller.

The Mental Approach

Fitness is no longer solely body-oriented; nowadays the emphasis is on the body and the mind. Yoga, tai chi, karate fessor of internal medicine and gerontology at the University of Washington School of Medicine in Seattle. Exercise doesn't just incinerate calories on the spot; it may also raise your metabolic rate, keeping it revving even after you stop exercising. The reward: You burn more calories at rest. You can still eat heartily (providing, of course, it's low-fat fare) because your body's metabolic motor is burning more fuel.

Beyond metabolic mastery, why is exercise potentially better than plain old dieting at targeting the midsection? "There may be something unique to exercise that creates a preferential weight loss," says Dr. Schwartz.

Exercise may stimulate growth-hormone secretion, which declines in older people. "It's fairly clear that when you give growth hormone to growth-hormone-deficient people, they gain lean mass and lose fat, especially abdominal fat," he says. "It's not clear right now, however, but activity may somehow prevent this age-related growth-hormone loss. That means holding on to muscle and blocking an increase in central body fat that occurs with aging."

and stretching have become mainstream. "People not only want to look good on the outside, they also want to feel good on the inside," says Evelyn Hamann, fitness director at RiverPlace Athletic Club in Portland, Oregon.

When Mirabai Holland started teaching her classes in the New York City area, she worried that aerobic-dance fanatics wired for high-impact classes wouldn't take to her softer, gentler approach. She didn't use music, and she didn't move quickly. Instead, her classes concentrated on breathing, body alignment and mental imagery. Turns out she had nothing to fear; hardbodies and first-time students welcomed her approach.

Ruth Stricker isn't surprised. Her latest research (conducted in conjunction with the University of Massachusetts and Harvard medical schools) shows that exercise combined with a cognitive strategy is superior to exercise alone in promoting psychological benefits. She defines fitness as being in "fighting shape" to combat whatever life has in store for you, whether it's daily stress, illness or aging. "It's time to turn fitness into wellness," says Kacy Duke, aerobics director at Equinox Fitness Club in New York City. "All of the emphasis shouldn't be on exercising and dieting to lose weight. Lifestyle changes need to promote a balance of mind, body and spirit."

The Next Wave

Water workouts have been making a splash, and for good reason: They are low-impact, safe, challenging and now—thanks to the new wave of water classes and the swanky pool props that go along with them—fun. "Aqua aerobics used to appeal only to older people, but my groups are getting younger and younger," says Mary Sanders, who founded Wave Aerobics in Reno, Nevada, ten years ago.

But beneath the surface, there's another reason for water's popularity: If you're not particularly well-coordinated, no one in your water aerobics class will know. "Doing aqua aerobics is like returning to the womb," says Steve Martin Mull, founder of Total Health in Saratoga, California. "We're suspended in fluid, we have the freedom to move around, and no one is there telling us if we're doing it right or wrong. It's as if you have your own little aerobics studio." Mull foresees a new wave of aqua gyms that focus exclusively on water workouts popping up across the country.

Reduce Seasonal Changes in Body Fat

If you notice your body's changing shape after winter and spring—don't get down on yourself, it's only as natural as the change in seasons. Researchers from Tufts University in Medford, Massachusetts, found that when they measured 125 women (using a whole-body scanner) over one year, older women may expect seasonal changes in their fat and lean mass even if they keep the same weight and activity levels throughout the year. These postmenopausal women had increases in muscle and bone mass during the summer/fall period and decreases during the winter/spring period. Their weights didn't change, though the women had a net loss of lean tissue in their legs and a net gain in fat tissue in their trunks.

But don't get bent out of shape: Even though these fluctuations had little to do with physical activity in this study, you can still use exercise to smooth them out, according to Bess Dawson-Hughes, M.D., from the U.S. Department of Agriculture Human Nutrition Research Center on Aging at Tufts, in Boston. "Even though the overall changes are consistent with what we've seen in body-shape changes due to the aging process, stepping up the exercise could help prevent many of the changes."

The loss of valuable muscle tissue (needed to perform essential daily functions), for example, could be reversed with walking and a few strength-training moves—a leg press or a partial squat. Tacking on a few extra walking sprees might help burn off some of the fat.

Dr. Dawson-Hughes hasn't figured out the reasons behind these seasonal fluctuations, but she speculates it may have to do with the brain's hypothalamus-pituitary area, which regulates several major hormones. "These hormones are known to influence those soft and hard tissues of the body."

The Family That Plays Together . . .

With Olympic gold medalist Florence Griffith Joyner at the helm, the President's Council on Physical Fitness and Sports has reshaped its focus to target the entire family. "The point of trying to improve children's fitness is to start them young," says council spokesman Phillip Wiethorn. "What better role model is there than the family?"

Is this a flashback to "Leave It to Beaver"? No, it's a reflection that exercisers today tend to share their passion with those closest to them. Hardworking parents see it as a way to spend time with the kids and still get in their exercise. Families have joined together to form cycling and running clubs; tennis tournaments that offer family doubles matches are springing up everywhere. Health clubs are beginning to add programs for kids. "Ten years ago, exercisers wanted to look good and attract the opposite sex," says Miller. "Now they have kids and want to make it past the age of 75. Exercise is no longer a life focus but part of the way to make life more balanced."

Even single men and women are searching for more family-style workouts. Miller reports that unmarried exercisers are joining together for group workouts, forcing her to differentiate between "private" one-to-one training and "personal" training, where several friends seeking common goals exercise together. Miller describes the trend this way: "*The Big Chill* has crept into the club."

—David Higdon

The Retreat That Refreshes

Rejuvenate body and soul at a restful getaway.

Our cup runneth over. That's midlife in a nutshell.
Our lives are overflowing with commitments and
decisions and problems and stresses. And if we're
filled to the brim, how can we ever expect to add
anything to enrich ourselves? "By the time we reach
midlife," says Stephan Rechtschaffen, M.D., director
of the Omega Institute, a retreat center in Rhine-
beck, New York, "we've accumulated so many commitments and responsibilities that we're just hanging
on, telling ourselves 'I can keep doing this till the
kids graduate' or 'until my next vacation.' We keep
plugging away despite the fact that many of our
habits are killing us."

The cost of being so busy and overwhelmed that
we disregard taking care of ourselves is great. Our
health suffers; our happiness dwindles; our spirits
sag. What we need, he says, is to find a way to
empty our proverbial cups, take some time for ourselves and create the opportunity for rejuvenation
and a fresh perspective.

One of the best ways to accomplish this is to literally plunk ourselves down in an entirely different,
refreshing environment void of the distractions of
work or home.

"Getting away, going on 'retreat,' affords a person a little time for himself," says Dr. Rechtschaffen. "In that time, you relax. You start to let go some and get empty. Only then can you begin to hear something new—something that's usually drowned out by the noise of everyday life."

Here are some of the rejuvenating elements you may find at a good retreat. Just remember that every element may not be present at every retreat, and some elements may suit your needs better than others.

A Slower Pace

The most important feature of a retreat is that it takes us out of our normal whirlwind pace and slows us down. "In the modern way of life, time is so sped up that most people suffer from the sensation of time urgency and anxiety," says Dr. Rechtschaffen, who leads weekend retreats called Time Shifting: Creating Time for Your Life and week-long retreats called the Omega Wellness Program. "People need to take what I call a time retreat, where they come into a period of time that's slowed down and different from that sense of rush."

The visual impact of slowing the pace is like "watching a flower open," he notes. "You see people who are anxious, worrying 'Are we going to get there on time? Do you have all my luggage?' and so on. And at the end of the week, they have smiles on their faces and color in their cheeks. They couldn't care less about the luggage!" Slowing our pace allows our cups to empty. It creates space internally into which new ideas and new possibilities for living can flow.

Education and Empowerment

Retreats afford people the opportunity to have a different type of education, one in which they're tuning in to themselves and learning what it is they really need in life, not what somebody else is saying they need or just continuing with the status quo.

"It's the chance to see what you've been doing and change it if necessary or reaffirm that that's how you want it to continue," says Dr. Rechtschaffen.

That's of utmost importance at midlife, when so many of us are re-evaluating our life's purpose and direction. "Retreats are a way of going deeper within ourselves as a way of re-evaluating what it is we want in our lives," he says. One fundamental goal of good education is empowerment: to help people understand what has brought them to certain lifestyle factors that contribute to their dissatisfaction or less-than-optimal health.

"People themselves can best discover what it is they need—whether it's to improve stress-management skills, to take more time for themselves, to make changes in diet or exercise or to get involved with a community," says Stephen Nezezon, M.D., a psychiatrist and staff physician at the Himalayan Institute in Honesdale, Pennsylvania. "We feel that a person is healthy only when he is able to manage his own health. Once a person has the background to understand what disease is and where it comes from and has acquired the tools to work effectively with his problem, then we feel that person is moving positively on the road to health."

Getting a retreat education can help provide us with those tools.

Time to Practice

The benefit of immersion in a retreat environment is that it facilitates actual changes in people's lives—not just changes in what they know. Retreats can help change your lifestyle from an unhealthy, unsatisfying one to one that's truly revitalizing. One reason that real changes can be made at a retreat is that it allows for a lengthy period of time to practice changes. People can participate in the changes and learn in a way that they can then go home and integrate into their lifestyles.

This practice is reinforced by an interactive environment in which people share their experiences and learn from each other. As a result, a supportive community develops. "Community is very nurturing," says Dr. Rechtschaffen. "The minute you feel real support from others, you drop your defenses. The creation of a safe environment allows people to change, to learn and to deepen."

Bodyworks

One of the best ways we can de-stress and rejuvenate ourselves is to get massages and other kinds of bodywork, an integral offering at many retreats.

"Being touched allows us to return to that childlike state of safety, where it's very much okay to be taken care of and nurtured," says Dana Bass Smith, director of Two Bunch Palms, a spa retreat center in Desert Hot Springs,

---

A Guide for Finding a Retreat

The Spa-Finders Worldwide Catalog of Spas, Fitness Resorts and Retreats. This full-size, glossy magazine includes specific information on a variety of types of spas and retreats. For ordering information, write to Spa-Finders, 91 Fifth Avenue, Suite 301, New York, NY 10003. For more information, call 1-800-255-7727.

California. "Touch can let the tensions of the body and mind release."

People of all ages, shapes and sizes sojourn to spas for rejuvenation in the warm-water soaks, daily massages and serene atmosphere. Midlifers often come when they're burned out and desperate for some tender loving care.

"If people can get over the initial risk and allow themselves to be touched and massaged, they will ultimately benefit from the experience," says Bass Smith.

Soothing Silence

Peace and quiet is a quality many seek in retreat. One of the reasons we so rarely experience peace and quiet in our daily lives is that culturally, we have a resistance to passivity.

"Americans need to learn how to sit and not be busy, not do anything," says Bruce Davis, Ph.D., a psychologist who leads silent retreats to Assisi, Italy, and author of *Monastery without Walls.*

"In silence, you learn that you can be passive and you don't have to manage everything," says Carol Wilkinson, director of Dayspring Silent Retreat Center, in Germantown, Maryland. "You learn to wait and listen and let be. Just because your action is diminished doesn't mean you are diminished."

Initially, turning down the volume on external noise brings all the chatter and thoughts going on inside our heads to the fore. "When we can't be with the silence, what we're really saying is that we can't be with ourselves," says Dr. Davis. "But if you sit with that chaos, breathe and let it go more and more, you come to a very quiet, peaceful place where you can deeply rest."

Ironically, what happens in restful silence is that people begin to hear. "As you cut down on external stimuli, inter-

(continued on page 232)

Profiles in Retreat Rejuvenation

Susan Goldberg, 40

In the early summer of 1992, my mother, who had been ill for about a year, started to decline. I was living in California and my parents were in Illinois, and I started making frequent trips home. There was some unresolved emotional conflict with my mother that was weighing upon me. So we had a couple of very intense visits, and fortunately, everything resolved beautifully. Somehow we were able to say everything we needed to say and tell each other we loved each other. It was incredible. The love and even joy were mixed in with the whole sad experience.

By midsummer, soon after I'd made two really intense trips within a month, my mother went into an even more rapid decline. I was quickly called back as she was dying. But my flight arrangements got mixed up, and I missed her by an hour or two.

Soon after returning to Los Angeles, I realized that I was emotionally exhausted and that what I craved was to be taken care of myself. I desperately needed to be touched and nurtured. I imagined being in a situation where I wouldn't have to put any energy out, where I could completely let go and not have to be in control. So I decided to spend five days at a spa.

Words can't describe how nurturing the environment felt right from the start. The desert oasis was dotted with palm trees and small hot-spring ponds, all under pure, deep-blue skies. There was a lush organic garden and a gurgling brook.

I stayed alone in a cute little cabinlike room and hardly spoke to anybody for five days. I spent almost all of my time getting massages and body 'treatments,' floating in the hot-spring pools and taking long walks on the lush grounds.

Even though most of the treatments were physical, involving massage and touch, they affected me emotionally as well.

One of my favorites was called the Roman Tub Rejuvenator. It started with a slow, deep massage for 45 minutes in a small outdoor gazebo. Next, I was led to a sweet-smelling aromatherapy bath in natural hot-spring water in a dark room lit with candles. I slipped deeper into relaxation as I enjoyed the fragrant steam.

After I had a long soak, the therapist took me back to the pavilion, gave me a final finishing massage, wrapped me in a warm blanket and left me lying there as the sun set and the birds sang. I felt like an infant being bathed and wrapped and laid in the crib.

And it was exactly what I needed—to be able to rest completely and fully. Allowing myself to have this nurturing experience helped me to realize my own strength. I realized that I was the one who had to supply myself with what was missing emotionally. I had to let go of whatever kind of need or false hope I had that I could get what I needed from someone else. Only then could I begin the deep-healing process.

Leighton Dorey, 48

The Monday after I turned 45, I had my annual physical exam. I felt fine, so you can imagine my surprise when my doctor came across a tender spot in my abdomen. Tests confirmed I had colon cancer.

My life went on hold. First I had surgery, then chemotherapy once a week for ten months. All my energy was channeled into making my body well. And yet I realized that my mental health needed healing, too.

Before I got sick, I was creating a high level of stress. My real-estate business was riding the boom of the 1980s. And my wife and I had undertaken a major renovation of an

(continued)

Profiles in Retreat Rejuvenation—
Continued

eighteenth-century farmhouse (with me as the general con-
tractor). I was running at breakneck speed, nonstop, 16 hours
a day.

When I found out I had cancer, I slammed on the brakes.

Determined not to overstress myself again, I decided to
follow my course of conventional cancer therapy with some
unconventional mind/body therapy. I signed up for a weekend introductory course on meditation at a retreat center.

I learned so much in those two days that I decided to
return for an intensive two-week program of stress reduction
and mind/body healing. The program was limited to six participants, many of whom had faced major illnesses.

Every day for an hour, I met with a physician and a psychiatrist. The three of us discussed my physical and emotional
well-being. We explored my attitudes about myself, my relationships with my family and my feelings about having cancer.

I also learned stress-management techniques and took
classes on exercise and diet. Each morning began with an
hour of hatha yoga. I used to think yoga was just a stretching
exercise. But it is much more than that. The purpose behind
it is to calm the mind and body. There is a continual emphasis on paying attention to the breath and breathing in time
with yoga movements. It produced a level of relaxation I had
never previously experienced in my life.

I also had a half-hour biofeedback session every morning
and afternoon. The purpose of biofeedback is to graphically
show you your body's stress response so you can learn to
induce relaxation.

The technician placed three electrodes on my forehead to
measure tension and on my fingers and thumbs to measure
body temperature, pulse rate and sweat. He put two bands

around my chest to measure my breathing. Then I watched a monitor that displayed exactly what my body was doing.

It's easy to raise your heart rate with a little excitement or exercise, but it's not as easy to lower it. With the help of the biofeedback readouts, I learned how to consciously raise and lower my heart rate and skin temperature.

One day, I came up for my biofeedback session, and the readings weren't good. I growled at the machine 'What are you doing producing numbers like this?' Then I laughed, realizing that all of these numbers were just a reflection of my hassled state. So as I had been instructed, I corrected my slumped posture, sat perfectly erect and started deep breathing from my diaphragm instead of my chest. Within two minutes, my tension readings on the machine dropped 50 percent!

Another activity that really broadened my horizons was chanting. The first time I was invited, I smiled politely but recoiled—'No, thank you!' Later, however, I decided to put aside my preconceptions and go to see what it was all about. What I heard was like a magnet drawing me in—very relaxing and almost mesmerizing.

Everyone in the audience was participating—singing and playing instruments. A girl up front with a beautiful voice would sing a stanza, and the audience would sing it back. Dispersed throughout the audience were tambourines, a flute and two sets of small drums, which anyone could play. The sound was all around, and it was a marvelously relaxing experience.

For me, the retreat experience wasn't just a quick fix. It was a learning experience in the truest sense; I learned by doing. This was a vacation, different from all the rest, in that it produced benefits for the rest of my life.

nal sensations begin to bubble up," says Wilkinson. "Dealing with emotions in silence can bring about an entirely different outcome, helping us forge new, better ways of being and relating."

Take anger as an example. "Instead of exploding," she says, "if you sit with anger in silence and listen to it, you can learn what your anger has to teach you about yourself. If you listen to it carefully, you may be surprised what you can learn about yourself. Your actions will be informed by a wisdom deeper than your own." Some people are drawn to attend retreats that are silent from start to finish. "Being in silence in community is very healing," says Wilkinson. "Social realities don't intrude. People who don't have to make conversation encounter each other at a different level." Many people find a spiritual dimension in the silence.

"It has a presence to it," says Dr. Davis. "Feeling that, we realize we're not alone, that we're part of something bigger, whether you call it God or whatever you want to call it. It feels like we connect to everything—to nature, to animals, to life—that we're related beyond our daily reality."

Taking the Plunge

Many people are reluctant to take time for themselves at a retreat because they think it's self-indulgent or selfish. "That's a common, though misguided, impediment," says Ross Goldstein, Ph.D., San Francisco psychologist and author of *Fortysomething*. "I remind people to think of the familiar safety instruction we always hear on airplanes: If the cabin should experience a loss of pressure, and the oxygen masks drop down, put your own mask on first before helping another person." The logic, he concludes, is clear. If you don't take care of yourself, you aren't going to be any good to anybody else.

—Sharon Stocker

Part Nine

Slash the Fat, Save the Flavor

Eating Light in the Real World

Best bets for on-the-go dieters.

You're cruising down the interstate when breakfast beckons. It's fast food or nothing, but can you refuel on such fare without taking a detour around your healthy diet?

You're spending an afternoon at the ballpark. Hunger strikes just as you catch a tantalizing whiff of hot dogs. A transgression can send your diet to the dugout, but can you resist?

Situations like these can be challenging for weight- and health-conscious people. But no matter how difficult a situation, choices are usually available—some better than others.

The key in these circumstances is to make choices actively, not passively, says Sachiko St. Jeor, Ph.D., professor of nutrition at the University of Nevada School of Medicine in Reno. "You don't have to be a victim of your environment," Dr. St. Jeor says. "You can take control."

Please Your Sweet Tooth without Fat

Sweet snacks and after-dinner TV watching go hand in hand. Problem is, most sweet munchies contain loads of calorie-laden fat. And while sugar won't necessarily spoil your diet, the fat that often accompanies it certainly will.

Sugar is a carbohydrate, akin to high-powered foods such as pastas, potatoes and beans, and is burned off quickly as energy. Dietary fat, on the other hand, contains twice as many calories per gram as sugar and is far more readily stored as flab.

The challenge, then, is to please your sweet tooth without indulging your fat fetish as well.

Our suggestion? Reach for your kid's cereal. Varieties such as Cap'n Crunch's Peanut Butter Crunch, which contains only three grams of fat per 120-calorie serving (under the cutoff of 25 percent of total calories), and Golden Crunch, which contains no fat, provide lots of sweetness. And because they're fortified, they contain healthful vitamins and minerals, too. Other good choices include Honey Nut Cheerios, Apple Jacks and Cinnamon Life.

With those words of inspiration in mind, we decided to explore some real diet danger zones to find good, better and best choices. Here are some ideas that may help you make informed food choices in any situation.

Fast-Food Breakfast

Good: Pancakes. A decent choice in any fast-food restaurant, assuming you hold the butter or margarine and go easy on the syrup. At Hardee's, which offers the most diet-friendly pancakes by fast-food standards, three cakes contain 280 calories and just two grams of fat (6 percent of calories). McDonald's pancakes aren't bad either, with 245 calories and four grams of fat (15 percent of calories) in three.

Better: McDonald's fat-free apple bran muffin. Only 180 calories, no fat. Add six ounces of orange juice (about 60 calories and no fat) and eight ounces of 1 percent milk (about 110 calories and two grams fat), and you have a pretty nutritious, low-fat breakfast for 350 calories, says Dr. St. Jeor.

Best: A bowl of nonsugary cereal. McDonald's serves up Cheerios (¾ cup for 80 calories and one gram fat) and Wheaties (¾ cup for 90 calories and one gram fat)—either of which provides about 15 to 30 percent of the Recommended Dietary Allowance (RDA) for vitamins A and C and iron. Pour on the 1 percent milk, and the total calorie count is still under 200—plus you meet about a third of your daily calcium requirement.

Fast-Food Chicken Sandwiches

Good: Arby's Lite Roast Chicken Deluxe or Wendy's Grilled Chicken Sandwich. Now, here are two sandwiches worth clucking about. Arby's has 276 calories and seven grams of fat (23 percent of calories). Wendy's chicken sandwich is close, with 290 calories and seven grams of fat (22 percent of calories).

Better: Chick-Fil-A Chargrilled Chicken Sandwich. This East Coast chain offers one lean chicken, with just 17 percent of calories from fat, 258 calories, 4.8 grams fat. If you have high blood pressure, however, take note: This sandwich may be low in fat, but it's high in sodium, with 1,121 milligrams.

Beware: A chicken sandwich by any other name could be a fat trap. Burger King's Chicken Sandwich, for example, will set you back 700 calories, with 54 percent of those calories from fat. McDonald's McChicken (470 calories and 25 grams fat), Wendy's Breaded Chicken (450 calories, 20 grams fat) and Arby's Grilled Chicken Deluxe sandwiches (430 calories, 19.9 grams fat) aren't much better, with about 40 to 48 percent of calories from fat. Squawk!

Cinema Fare

Okay: Red licorice. Red Vines, for example, by American Licorice Company, has only 140 calories and zero fat in seven five-inch red licorice sticks. Trouble is, we're talking empty calories here; red licorice has virtually no nutrient value.

Better: Nonbuttered popcorn. Only 55 calories, about 100 milligrams sodium and about 3.1 grams of fat per cup for oil-popped corn—plus it provides approximately one gram of fiber per cup. The problem is, most theaters serve up popcorn by the gallon, and few people can stop at a cup, which makes fat, calorie and sodium totals soar.

Best: Eat before the film. "Remind yourself that movies last just two hours, and you can go that long without food," says Dr. St. Jeor. "Get into watching the movie as a pure experience, without shoveling down food you can't see or really enjoy."

Airport Food

Good: Sushi. It's becoming as all-American as bagels. In airports, stick with the kind with the cooked fish filling (like those with crabmeat) or vegetable filling to avoid risk of parasites, says *Prevention* advisor Judith S. Stern, R.D.,

When Low-Calorie Isn't

Those "low-calorie" brownies and cookies may be lighter in the truth than they are in calories.

Looking at the goods under 40 foods with "diet" and "health food" labels, researchers found that calorie counts were underreported by as much as 85 percent. Laboratory tests showed national brands to be straight about calories, but not so with smaller or local brands. Regionally distributed foods (ones packaged by the neighborhood grocery store or not distributed on a national scale) packed an average of 25 percent more calories than the labels claimed. Local products, made by neighborhood restaurants or candy stores, were way off, holding up to 85 percent more calories than what was advertised.

"We expected large companies had the facilities and the wherewithal to be accurate, and they were," says study author David B. Allison, Ph.D., research fellow at the Obesity Research Center at St. Luke's–Roosevelt Hospital in New York City. The smaller companies' inaccuracies may have been due to poor testing, he says. These companies may have a difficult time getting to (and paying for) the best calorie-testing equipment.

Until labels are more standard, keep your healthy eating on track by planning around that extra 85 percent— consider counting that 100-calorie brownie as 185 calories. Or be on the safe side and use foods that don't need labels that tout health claims. With foods like beans, grains, fruits, vegetables, lean meats and fish, you know what you're getting.

Sc.D., a nutrition professor at the University of California, Davis. A full serving of vegetable sushi contains about 365 calories and just one gram fat.

Better: Nonfat frozen yogurt. Four ounces of Honey Hill Farms' Ghirardelli Chocolate flavor, for example, contains 115 calories, no fat and, as a bonus, 110 milligrams of calcium—a boon for the bones. (Skip the "mix-ins" like chopped candy and nuts.)

Even better: A steaming cup of decaf café latte (made with skim milk). A café latte is mostly hot milk, with a little espresso floated on top. You sate your appetite and do your bones a favor calciumwise (264 milligrams in seven ounces for less than 80 calories and less than ½ gram of fat).

Best: Don't let boredom ignite your appetite—take a fitness walk through the terminal. You can chart your course and ensure that you don't get lost by picking up a map of the terminal at the information desk. Many airports also have lockers where you can stash your carry-ons. Tip: Wear a fanny pack or backpack so you can stride more freely in your travels.

Burgers in Disneyland

Good: Turkey Burger. Served with lettuce, tomato and fat-free Thousand Island dressing on a honey wheat bun, it has 367 calories and 9.5 grams of fat (23 percent of calories).

Best: Veggie Burger. Same fat-free dressing and bun, with only 365 calories and eight grams of fat (20 percent of calories).

Mixed Drinks

Good: Virgin (nonalcoholic) fresh-fruit daiquiris. About 80 to 100 calories, with little or no fat. The standard recipe calls for about ½ cup of fresh fruit (like strawberries, which contain roughly 30 calories plus some fiber and vitamin C), two ounces of a mixer called sweet and sour (a nonfat lemon-and-sugar drink, with about 50 calories for two ounces) and a big scoop of ice.

Best: Virgin Mary. This spicy tomato-juice concoction is a boon to the weight-conscious in so many ways. It fills you with liquid; it's low-cal—about 32 calories for a six-ounce glass—with no fat; it's spicy, which satisfies taste buds; it provides some nutrition in the form of vitamin C; and finally, there's a great big celery stick to provide crunch appeal.

Ballpark Fare

Good: Check out the latest offerings. It's a whole new ball game out there! Stadium concessionaires are innovating to appeal to the increasing numbers of female sports fans, says Matthew Bauer, media manager for Sportservice Corporation in Buffalo, New York, the leading food supplier to ballparks across the country. Among the new offerings:

- Rotisserie chicken, an alternative to fried chicken, available at Texas Rangers Stadium in Arlington, Texas. (A great choice, as long as you remove the skin!) Also in several parks: grilled chicken served on a bed of greens.
- The vegetarian burrito at Tiger Stadium in Detroit, loaded with julienned strips of zucchini, peppers and onions in a soft flour tortilla.
- Fresh sliced-turkey sandwiches at Dodger Stadium in Los Angeles and other locales.
- Frozen-fruit pops, along with low-fat frozen yogurt, as an alternative to ice cream, available at Sportservice client stadiums, including Milwaukee County Stadium, Riverfront Stadium in Cincinnati, Comiskey Park in Chicago, Busch Stadium in St. Louis and Gateway Stadium in Cleveland.

Best: Crudités. At Dodger Stadium, they give it a more manly name (relish tray), but that's what it is—a plate loaded with fresh cucumbers, celery, carrots and radishes.

Beware: "In-your-seat" service. A less-fortunate new trend in stadium cuisine is the legion of waiters sent out with handheld computers who take your order at your seat and then deliver it to you. Just say no! Stand up and go get it yourself! Walking burns calories!

Chinese Meals

Good: A shared entrée of stir-fried vegetables and lots of steamed rice. Chinese-food lovers reeled in shock when news stories revealed that many of our favorite dishes are loaded with fatty oils. And it's true: A typical serving of stir-fried veggies can contain 400 calories and anywhere from 6 to 18 grams of fat. But you can avoid some of the fat and still enjoy this flavorful cuisine by sharing an entrée. To appease your appetite, pile on the steamed rice.

Best: Steamed veggies with chicken or shrimp. Even if it's not on the menu, most cooks in Chinese restaurants know how and have what it takes to create a delectable steamed meal. Often, they serve it in a beautiful bamboo steamer. For flavor, sprinkle with soy sauce or ask for a brown sauce with scallions on the side to drizzle on top. In these entrées, light-meat chicken contains only about 175 calories and 5 grams of fat, while shrimp is even leaner, with only about 22 calories and a skimpy ¼ gram fat.

Restaurant Desserts

Good: Two or more forks, so you can share dessert with a friend—or the whole table. "If you're used to eating dessert and you let yourself have just a bite or two, you'll be less likely to feel deprived and binge later," says John Foreyt, Ph.D., a nutrition professor at Baylor College of Medicine in Houston and author of *Living without Dieting*.

Better: Decaf cappuccino. Have a decaf cappuccino (espresso with frothed skim milk) served with a biscotti or two on the side, suggests nutritionist Evelyn Tribole, R.D., spokesperson for the American Dietetic Association and author of *Eating on the Run*. Many different companies are manufacturing biscotti, which are almond dipping cookies. They're generally low in fat and calories, though counts do vary. We've seen some biscotti with a respectable 30 calories and less than one gram of fat per cookie.

Best: Sorbet. This tangy fruit-juice-based dessert is mostly water. One-half cup of fruit sorbet, such as pineapple or peach, might provide about 120 calories and no fat, plus a handy 12 milligrams of vitamin C.

Chocolate Lovers' Supermarket Snacks

Good: Snack Well's Devil's Food Cookie Cakes. Deep chocolate, cakey interior surrounded by a thin layer of marshmallow, then a dark chocolate coating—so sweet and rich, it's hard to believe they're fat-free. Drawbacks: Each hefty cookie contains about 50 calories, so you can't eat infinite amounts. They don't really offer vitamins or minerals, either. And the leading ingredient is sugar.

Special mention: Chocolate-flavored low-fat yogurt. Would you believe chocolate raspberry yogurt? Chocolate cherry? Chocolate cappuccino? They're really, really chocolaty and contain only 200 calories for ¾ cup, with just two grams of fat but 20 percent of the RDA for calcium. They're put out by Whitney's of New York. Unfortunately, they're not available everywhere yet—they're being test-marketed in Baltimore, Washington, D.C., and Pennsylvania. We're hoping they become a national trend soon.

Seafood Entrées

Good: Haddock. Just 112 calories and about one gram of fat (8 percent of calories) for 3½ ounces.

Best: Lobster. The winner and still champion. Steamed

or boiled, it gets just 5.4 percent calories from fat. Three and one-half ounces of lobster meat contains less than one gram of fat and just 98 calories. You'll need to skip the melted butter, however—try cocktail sauce instead.

Beware: Tuna salad. Sorry, Charlie. A cup of tuna salad, with regular mayo, provides 380 calories and 19 grams of fat (45 percent of calories).

Munchies

Good: Crisp baked Bugles. We didn't believe it till we tried them ourselves. Unlike the regular Bugles product (with 150 calories and eight grams of fat for every serving), the kind marked "oven-baked" is relatively low-calorie (90 calories for 42 Bugles) and low-fat (two grams fat). But like the regular product, the oven-baked Bugles taste oily and crunchy. (Sodium's pretty high, though, at 300 milligrams per serving, and they don't offer many nutrients.)

Better: Air-popped popcorn. Three cups contains only 93 calories and a gram of fat, plus about three grams fiber.

Better yet: Fat-free (baked) potato chips or tortilla chips. Guiltless Gourmet No-Oil Tortilla Chips contain 110 calories for 22 chips, a respectable four grams of fiber plus 10 percent of the RDA for calcium—and zero fat. Similarly, Louise's Fat Free Potato Chips contain about 100 calories per ounce, no fat and 10 percent of the RDA for vitamin C.

Beef

Good: Healthy Choice Extra Lean Low-Fat Ground Beef. Four ounces (uncooked) contains 4 grams fat—that's about 28 percent of its calories. By comparison, four ounces of regular ground beef contains 30 grams fat (that's 77 percent of calories from fat).

Better: Select-grade top and eye round. With about 20

to 25 percent of calories from fat, this is a cut above all other supermarket-grade cuts.

Best: New brands of beef that are raised to be low in fat through diet. We've heard of several, like Dakota Lean Meats. Most of the Dakota cuts—ranging from top sirloin to tenderloin to sirloin tips—average about 2.7 grams fat and 130 calories for every four-ounce serving. That's a respectable 19 percent of calories from fat. Ask your butcher.

—Cathy Perlmutter with Linda Rao and Teresa Yeykal

A Taste of Summer

Toss garden-fresh greens with grilled meats for lean, luscious flavor.

Try a summer salad from the grill. It's so easy. All you do is take your favorite dinner fixings—dark leafy greens, vine-ripened tomatoes, fresh veggies and perhaps a little lean meat or seafood that's been grilled or roasted to perfection—and assemble them in an artful presentation drizzled with a simple dressing. The beauty of grilled salads is that they offer exciting new taste sensations. In effect, the whole is much better—and more delicious—than the sum of its parts. Just as traditional hot dressings partially warm and wilt the greens they adorn, hot grilled foods interact wonderfully with robust greens. And warm foods tend to absorb dressing, making them even more flavorful.

This concept of mixing greens and dinner fixings is so elementary that you don't actually need a recipe. But we've created four just to get you started.

GRILLED SALMON AND FENNEL SALAD

This salad is lovely, combining the pink color of the fish with the green of the fennel and the purple of red onions. For variety, you can easily substitute any other type of seafood, including shrimp, scallops or firm-fleshed fish. The potatoes make this salad quite substantial. Although we've given directions for roasting the potatoes on the grill, you can easily cut leftover baked potatoes into thick slabs and place them on the hot grill just long enough to heat them through and score them with attractive grill marks.

    4 medium potatoes (1 pound total)
    4 small fennel bulbs
    8 ounces salmon fillet
    1 large tomato, peeled, seeded and chopped
    ¼ cup chopped red onions
    1 small sweet red pepper, chopped
    3 tablespoons balsamic vinegar
    1 tablespoon olive oil
    1 clove garlic, chopped
    ¼ teaspoon ground black pepper
    1 cup tender spinach leaves

Scrub the potatoes and wrap them individually in foil. If using charcoal or wood chips, bury the potatoes among the hot coals; if using a gas grill, place the potatoes directly on the grids. Grill about 40 to 45 minutes, or until easily pierced with a knife.

Cut the feathery tops from the fennel, reserving some for a garnish. Quarter the bulbs lengthwise. Discard any tough outer leaves. Steam for 10 minutes, or until still slightly crunchy. (Test with a knife tip.) Rinse carefully under cold water and set aside.

Place the salmon on the grill and cook it for 15 to 20 minutes, or until done as you prefer it. Place the fennel on the grill and cook briefly until striped on two sides and heated through.

While the salmon is grilling, place the tomatoes, onions, red peppers, vinegar, oil, garlic and black pepper in a blender or food processor. Process with on/off turns until finely chopped but still a little chunky.

Divide the spinach leaves among 4 dinner plates. Cut the salmon fillet into 4 portions and place on the plates. Unwrap the potatoes, cut into chunks and place on the plates. Add the grilled fennel. Drizzle with the dressing. If desired, garnish with reserved fennel greens. Serve at room temperature or chilled.

Serves 4.

Per serving: 287 calories, 7.8 g. fat (24% of calories), 7.6 g. dietary fiber, 17.1 g. protein, 40 g. carbohydrates, 31 mg. cholesterol, 206 mg. sodium. Also a very good source of niacin, vitamin A, vitamin B_6, vitamin B_{12}, vitamin C and potassium.

LAMB AND GREEN BEAN SALAD

You don't need much protein to serve a filling and satisfying dinner. Here, eight ounces of lamb is sufficient for four people because the meat is combined with beans, greens and hearty peasant-type bread. If you have access to fresh rosemary, throw some wet sprigs on the grill to help perfume the lamb as it cooks. If lamb isn't to your liking, substitute boneless, skinless chicken breasts, pounded to about ⅓-inch thickness before grilling, so they cook evenly. Or for a completely vegetarian meal, try portobello mushrooms instead.

> 8 **ounces small green beans, boiled for 5 minutes and drained**
> 8 **ounces lamb (lean)**
> 2 **cloves garlic, halved**
> 7 **thick slices rustic bread, divided**
> 2½ **teaspoons olive oil, divided**
> 3 **tablespoons red wine vinegar**
> 2 **ounces goat cheese, at room temperature**
> 2 **tablespoons lemon juice**
> 2 **tablespoons fat-free mayonnaise**
> 1 **tablespoon chopped walnuts**
> 1 **teaspoon minced fresh rosemary**
> 4 **ounces mesclun, watercress, arugula or other salad greens**

Using a skewer, poke some holes in a square of heavy-duty aluminum foil; place the beans on the foil and set aside.

Rub both sides of the lamb with 1 garlic half and set aside.

Cut 6 of the bread slices in half. Using ½ teaspoon of the oil, lightly brush the top of each. Then sprinkle the bread with 1 tablespoon of the vinegar.

Grill the lamb, green beans (on the foil) and bread until the lamb is done to taste, the beans are tender and the bread is golden on both sides. Remove from the grill.

Lightly rub the bread with the remaining cut cloves of garlic. Spread with the goat cheese. Cut the lamb into bite-size pieces. Remove the crust from the remaining slice of bread. Tear the bread into pieces, place in a blender and process into crumbs. Add the lemon juice, mayonnaise, walnuts, remaining 2 teaspoons oil and remaining 2 tablespoons vinegar. Puree until smooth. Stir in the rosemary.

Divide the greens among 4 dinner plates. Add the lamb and beans. Drizzle with the dressing. Serve with the bread.

Serves 4.

Per serving: 337 calories, 8.5 g. fat (23% of calories), 2.7 g. dietary fiber, 23.1 g. protein, 40.5 g. carbohydrates, 47 mg. cholesterol, 448 mg. sodium. Also a very good source of vitamins A and C.

TENDER PORK SALAD

Thinly sliced pieces of pork tenderloin cook quickly on the grill and go beautifully with grilled peppers, mushrooms and eggplant. These ingredients are particularly good served fajita-style in warm corn tortillas. For extra measure, you can grill fresh corn on the cob and serve it along with the meat and other vegetables.

    1   tablespoon low-sodium soy sauce
    2   cloves garlic, minced
    4   teaspoons chopped fresh oregano or marjoram,
        divided
    5½ teaspoons olive oil
    8   ounces pork tenderloin
    ½   cup lemon juice
    1   pound large mushrooms, thickly sliced
    2   sweet red peppers, thickly sliced
    2   green peppers, thickly sliced
    2   Japanese eggplants, quartered lengthwise
    4   ears corn, shucked and boiled for 3 minutes
    8   cups mixed bitter greens
    ¼   teaspoon ground black pepper
    12 corn tortillas

In a large bowl, mix the soy sauce, garlic, 1 teaspoon of the oregano or marjoram and 1 teaspoon of the oil. Add the pork and turn to coat all sides. Allow to marinate for 30 minutes.

In a small bowl, mix the lemon juice, the remaining 3 teaspoons oregano or marjoram and the remaining 4½ teaspoons of oil. Set aside.

Place a wire mesh screen over the grill rack. Add the mushrooms, red peppers, green peppers and eggplant pieces. Cut the corn ears into 2-inch sections and place on the grill. Grill for 5 to 10 minutes, then flip the pieces, using long-handled tongs, and grill for another 5 minutes, or until cooked as desired. Remove to a platter.

When the vegetables are nearly done, cut the pork cross-wise into 8 slices. Add to the grill and cook for 2 minutes per side, or until just cooked through. Divide the greens among 4 dinner plates. Top with the pork and vegetables. Sprinkle with the black pepper. Whisk the dressing and drizzle over the salads.

Wrap the tortillas in foil and warm in the coals for a few minutes. Serve with the salad. (If desired, eat the salad fajita-style.)

Serves 4.

Per serving: 498 calories, 13.1 g. fat (24% of calories), 16.8 g. dietary fiber, 27 g. protein, 77.5 g. carbohydrates, 37 mg. cholesterol, 369 mg. sodium. Also a very good source of thiamine, riboflavin, niacin, folate, vitamin A, vitamin B₆, vitamin C, iron, magnesium and potassium.

GRILLED CHICKEN WITH ZUCCHINI SALAD

This is really low in calories! And it's a nice way to serve tender young zucchini, which are cut into fan shapes and grilled to give them a smoky taste. As with most grilled salads, this one can be eaten hot, warm or chilled. Because cold foods tend to need more seasoning than warm ones, retaste chilled salads to see if they need a splash more vinegar.

2 boneless, skinless chicken breast halves (4 ounces each)
6 small thin zucchini (1½ pounds total)
1 medium Bermuda onion, sliced crosswise
2 tablespoons Pommery or other coarse mustard
2 tablespoons red wine vinegar
1 teaspoon olive oil
¼ cup minced fresh parsley
¼ teaspoon ground black pepper

Place the chicken between sheets of wax paper and pound to an even thickness of about ⅓ inch. Coat lightly with no-stick spray and set aside.

Cut each zucchini in half lengthwise. Cut each half lengthwise into thin strips, leaving the pieces attached at the stem end so that each piece becomes a fan.

Grill the chicken, zucchini and onions for 10 to 15 minutes, or until the chicken is cooked through, the zucchini is just tender and the onions are limp. Remove from the grill.

In a small bowl, whisk together the mustard, vinegar and oil. Stir in the parsley and pepper. Cut the grilled onion slices in half and add the strips to the bowl.

Cut the chicken into slices. Divide among 4 dinner plates. Add the zucchini strips and drizzle with the dressing.

Serves 4.

Per serving: 121 calories, 3.0 grams fat (22% of calories), 3.3 g. dietary fiber, 16 g. protein, 8.7 g. carbohydrates, 33 milligrams cholesterol, 145 mg. sodium. Also a very good source of niacin.

Building the Best Salad

Use these recipes as inspiration for your own summer salads from the grill. Below are considerations for each of the basic components as well as some practical tips. (For salad-dressing suggestions, see "Simple Low-Fat Dressings" on page 255.)

Greens. Sturdy greens like watercress, kale, radicchio, arugula, mustard greens, turnip greens, spinach, chard and beet greens (which also happen to be the most nutritious of the leafy greens) hold up well when mixed with warm ingredients. Fragile leaf lettuce doesn't fare as well. Certain types of greens can even be cooked right on the grill. Cut firm heads of Belgian endive, radicchio or romaine lengthwise into halves or quarters and place them on the grill rack for a few minutes per side, until lightly cooked and scored with grill marks.

Vegetables. Most types of vegetables are suitable for grilling. White potatoes, sweet potatoes, fennel, eggplant, peppers, onions, mushrooms, corn on the cob and zucchini give good results.

You can even do smaller items, like green beans and snap peas, if you use the following technique: Punch holes in a piece of heavy-duty aluminum foil, place it on the grill rack and scatter the vegetables over it. You'll get the smoky grill taste without worrying about the pieces ending up in the coals.

For variety in texture and flavor, toss a few raw veggies on your salad, too. A couple fresh tomato wedges or minis, like yellow pear tomatoes, or cucumber slices can add a delightful touch.

Meat, fish or seafood. Choose lean and tender cuts of beef, pork and lamb that will cook quickly on the grill. Tenderloin is the preferable cut, whether it's grilled as thinly sliced cutlets or whole as a roast and then sliced before serving.

Boneless, skinless chicken breasts are also perfect for grilling. Pound them to an even thickness first for even cooking.

You could also use boneless, skinless thighs; trim off as much visible fat as possible, then open up the pieces so they lie flat on the grill. Turkey tenders and sliced boneless, skinless turkey breast pieces are ideal for grilling, too.

When preparing fish, choose firm-fleshed types that don't fall apart on the grill. Swordfish, tuna, bluefish, grouper, monkfish, halibut, mako shark, salmon, mahi-mahi, snapper and sea bass are good. Use fillets, steaks or cubed pieces that you've threaded onto skewers.

The best way to grill shrimp and scallops is also on skewers. (If using bamboo or wooden skewers, soak them in cold water for at least 20 minutes first so they won't burn on the grill.) You could also use a mesh insert that fits right over your grill's grids to hold small pieces and prevent them from falling through.

And for added interest when grilling meat, fish or poultry, toss dried herb branches on the hot coals to help give food a little extra flavor.

Assembly. You can build beautiful salad arrangements on individual plates and easily make them look as elegant as any restaurant's.

If you're entertaining, use the occasion to do up a really elegant platter, in the manner of an antipasto, so your guests can serve themselves. (Cut a garlic clove or two in half and thoroughly rub the bottom and sides of the dish first to impart extra seasoning.)

No matter which serving option you choose, you can drizzle the dressing over the salad before laying the grilled vegetables or meats on top. Or place the dressing in a gravy boat or cruet and let diners add as much or little to their salads as they prefer.

Simple Low-Fat Dressings

When you're serving a very flavorful main-dish salad, you don't need to get fancy with the dressing. In fact, you can make a nice dressing from just the grilling juices that accumulate on the platter after you remove meat, fish, poultry or vegetables from the heat. Enhance them with a few drops of vinegar or a squeeze of lemon juice, a bit of garlic and some minced fresh herbs. Other easy ideas:

- Mash a garlic clove into a paste in a mortar, then blend with ¼ teaspoon mustard and a few grinds of black pepper from a pepper mill. Add vinegar and olive oil to taste.
- Grill a sweet red pepper until soft; discard the seeds. Puree the flesh with a clove of garlic, nonfat or reduced-fat cholesterol-free mayonnaise, a bit of tomato juice and a splash of vinegar.
- Another use for a grilled pepper: Puree it with roasted tomato halves (use equal amounts) and flavor with balsamic vinegar.
- Whisk together some rice-wine vinegar, a splash of sesame oil, minced fresh coriander and a drop or two of hot-pepper sauce.
- Mix the juice of an orange with a tablespoon of tomato paste. Flavor with fennel seeds, minced garlic and a pinch of powdered saffron.
- Take spicy salsa and thin it with some vinegar and a touch of oil.
- For the simplest of all dressings, just sprinkle on some full-bodied balsamic vinegar.

Alternatives to Outdoor Grilling

Cook meats or fish on a stove-top grill pan. A ridged cast-iron pan gives the same luscious-looking grill marks as a barbecue.

Oven-roast the vegetables. Cut potatoes, carrots, zucchini or other vegetables into uniform wedges or chunks, place on a no-stick baking sheet, drizzle with a bit of olive oil, if desired, and bake at 375° until well-browned on both sides—usually about 30 to 40 minutes.

The vegetables can be in the oven while the entrée is cooking on the stove.

If You Prefer a Meatless Meal

Huge portobello mushrooms make an excellent substitute for the meat in our Lamb and Green Bean Salad—or in any grilled salad, for that matter. They have a wonderfully meaty taste and texture.

Remove the stems, brush the caps with oil and place them on the grill, flat side down. When grill marks appear, give the mushrooms a quarter turn to add diagonal stripes. Then flip and roast until the edges are crisp. Cut into thin slices to serve.

New Life for Leftovers

Leftovers can make handy additions to a grilled salad. Try combining cold cooked pasta with grilled zucchini, eggplant or other vegetables, for instance. Or toss leftover rice (white, brown or wild) with grilled cubes of swordfish, bluefish or scallops and red or yellow peppers.

Add Grill Flavor to Classic Salads

Imagine how much better tabbouleh would be if you placed the cooked bulgur in a metal colander and then gave it a few minutes on the grill before adding the rest of the ingredients. (Cover the colander with foil to trap the smoky flavor.)

For extra measure, halve firm plum tomatoes and grill them until soft; let cool, then mix with the bulgur, parsley, mint, lemon juice and oil that characterize tabbouleh.

—*Judith Olney, Jean Rogers and Barb Fritz*

Blue-Ribbon Specials

Get a taste of the award-winning dishes from
Prevention *magazine's Healthy Recipe Contest*
winners.

Entries for this year's Healthy Recipe Contest topped out at over 14,000 recipes. Mark Bricklin and his trusted staff at the Rodale Food Center had the tasty task of sampling the fare.

They sipped their way through appetizers, dove into desserts and munched through many entrées, all in an effort to find this year's champions. Here are the winners.

Make It with Tuna

SPONSORED BY STAR-KIST NATURALLY LOW-SALT, LOW-FAT CHUNK TUNA

First Prize (in category) and Grand Prize overall: Priscilla Yee, Concord, California

For all the tuna lovers out there, here's an exotic-tasting dish you just have to try! Even if you're not a tuna lover, this dish is delicious. And it's ever so easy to make!

Priscilla, a tuna lover herself, cooked up this recipe because she was looking for a new way to serve tuna as a main dish.

The 45-year-old accountant for Pacific Bell finds her love for cooking "a way to come home and do something completely different from work, a way to relax."

Priscilla became interested in healthy cooking about 16 years ago, after her father had a heart attack. "I gradually changed my cooking over time so that this recipe is typical of the way I cook now," she says.

If this recipe is any indication of Priscilla's efforts at healthy cooking, she's doing very well. With only 23 percent of calories from fat, this dish is heart healthy and high in vitamins A and C.

When she's not working or cooking, Priscilla can be found at her company gym. The aerobics class is her favorite. On weekends, she enjoys walking and gardening.

TAHITIAN TUNA CAKES WITH GINGER SAUCE AND PAPAYA SALSA

GINGER SAUCE
>   1 cup nonfat yogurt
>   2 tablespoons lime juice
>   1 tablespoon grated fresh ginger
>   1 tablespoon coarse-grain mustard
>   2 teaspoons canola oil
>   ½ teaspoon ground cumin

PAPAYA SALSA
>   1½ cups cubed papaya
>   ½ cup chopped sweet red peppers
>   2 tablespoons chopped fresh cilantro
>   1 tablespoon lime juice
>   1 tablespoon honey
>   ¼ teaspoon ground red pepper

TUNA CAKES
>   2 cans (6⅛ ounces each) Star-Kist Naturally Low-Salt, Low-Fat Chunk Tuna, drained and flaked
>   ½ cup fat-free egg substitute
>   ¼ cup chopped scallions
>   1 cup fine dry bread crumbs, divided
>   1 tablespoon canola oil
>   Fresh cilantro sprigs (garnish)

To make the ginger sauce: In a small bowl, whisk together the yogurt, lime juice, ginger, mustard, oil and cumin. Set aside.

To make the papaya salsa: In a small bowl, mix the papaya, sweet peppers, cilantro, lime juice, honey and ground pepper. Set aside.

To make the tuna cakes: In a large bowl, combine the tuna, egg substitute, scallions, ⅔ cup of the bread crumbs and ¼ cup of the ginger sauce. Mix well. Shape into four ½-inch-thick patties. Coat with the remaining ⅓ cup bread crumbs.

In a large no-stick skillet over medium heat, warm the oil. Add the patties and sauté for 3 minutes per side, or until golden brown.

Transfer to individual plates. Drizzle with the remaining ginger sauce. Serve with the salsa and garnish with the cilantro.

Serves 4.

Per serving: 343 calories, 8.7 g. fat (23% of calories), 1.8 g. dietary fiber, 32.8 g. protein, 36.3 g. carbohydrates, 36 mg. cholesterol, 385 mg. sodium. Also a very good source of vitamins A and C.

Second Prize: Julie DeMatteo, Clementon, New Jersey

Julie originally made this recipe with steak, but since she and her husband, Nick, have cut back on red meat, she substituted tuna. Now they enjoy this scrumptious meal without the added fat.

TUNA BUNDLES DIABLO

 1 **scallion**
 1 **teaspoon canola oil**
 1 **clove garlic, minced**
 1 **can (6⅛ ounces) Star-Kist Naturally Low-Salt, Low-Fat Chunk Tuna, drained and flaked**
 ½ **cup cooked chopped spinach, well-drained**
 1 **tablespoon fine dry bread crumbs**
 ¼ **teaspoon ground black pepper**
 ½ **cup chunky salsa, divided**
 6 **sheets (12 × 17 inches each) phyllo dough**

Cut the dark green top from the scallion and slit the leaves in half lengthwise to make long ties; set aside. Finely chop the white and light green parts.

In a medium no-stick skillet, warm the oil over medium-high heat. Add the scallions and garlic. Sauté for 1 minute. Stir in the tuna and spinach and mix well. Add the bread crumbs, pepper and 2 tablespoons of the salsa. Remove from the heat and set aside.

Place 1 sheet of the phyllo on a clean, dry surface. (Keep the remaining sheets from drying out by covering them with a sheet of plastic wrap and a layer of damp paper towels.)

Coat the surface of the sheet with no-stick spray and fold it in half lengthwise. Place half of the tuna mixture near a 6-inch edge, centering it crosswise on the folded sheet. Fold in the long sides to cover the tuna, then roll up the strip to make a bundle. Repeat with a second sheet of phyllo and the remaining tuna to form another bundle. Set both aside.

Lay a third sheet of phyllo flat on the work surface and coat with no-stick spray. Cover with another sheet and spray. Place 1 of the rolled bundles in the center of the sheets.

Gather up the phyllo around the bundle, gently pressing it together in the center to form a sack. Take a long scallion top and gently tie it around the middle to hold the bundle together; be careful not to tear the scallion. Repeat with the remaining 2 sheets of phyllo and the second bundle.

Coat a baking sheet with no-stick spray. Place the bundles on the sheet and coat the tops and sides with no-stick spray. Bake at 400° for 15 to 20 minutes, or until golden brown.

Warm the remaining salsa in a small saucepan. Serve with the bundles.

Serves 2.

Per serving: 354 calories, 9.3 g. fat (24% of calories), 1.4 g. dietary fiber, 28.9 g. protein, 41 g. carbohydrates, 35 mg. cholesterol, 721 mg. sodium. Also a very good source of vitamin A.

Third Prize: Wendy K. Leece, West Bend, Wisconsin

This light and lemony side dish was the result of Wendy's addiction to lemons, her husband's love of couscous and the abundance of canned tuna they always have on hand in their pantry.

LEMON TUNA COUSCOUS

1 tablespoon olive oil
1 large onion, diced
2 cups shredded spinach leaves
5 cloves garlic, minced
1 can (6⅛ ounces) Star-Kist Naturally Low-Salt, Low-Fat Chunk Tuna, drained and flaked
½ teaspoon grated lemon peel
Juice of 1 lemon
1½ cups cooked couscous
2 tablespoons chopped fresh parsley
2 tablespoons grated Parmesan cheese
½ teaspoon ground black pepper

In a large no-stick skillet over medium heat, warm the oil. Add the onions, spinach and garlic and sauté for 3 minutes.

Reduce the heat to low. Add the tuna, lemon peel and lemon juice. Stir for a few minutes to heat through. Stir in the couscous, parsley, Parmesan and pepper and reheat.

Serves 2.

Per serving: 400 calories, 10.5 g. fat (24% of calories), 9.4 g. dietary fiber, 33.5 g. protein, 47.3 g. carbohydrates, 40 mg. cholesterol, 227 mg. sodium. Also a very good source of folate and vitamins A and C.

Make It an American Favorite

SPONSORED BY CRISCO PURITAN OIL
First Prize (in category) and First Runner-Up Grand Prize: Judy Koenig, Seattle, Washington

This recipe is a nutritional powerhouse! It's loaded with fiber, beta-carotene, vitamin C and much more!

One tester called it "Heavenly! I don't know how you could top this dish for nutrition or taste!"

For years, we've touted kale as a low-fat source of calcium. Now here's a great-tasting, easy way to add more kale to your diet.

We are fortunate to have this recipe, since Judy admits to never writing down recipes. "I just put things together; one time it will come out one way, and another time it will be a little bit different," she says.

While teaching English at a high school, Judy started cooking classes in an effort to educate her students on healthy eating and nutrition. What intensified her interest in healthy cooking? Perhaps it was the abundance of vegetables in her garden.

In addition to cooking, Judy enjoys yoga, walking, hiking and backpacking. She has also expanded her gardening into rose breeding and the development of a Chinese garden.

SOUTHERN BRAISED GREENS

    2 large sweet potatoes
    2 tablespoons Crisco Puritan Oil
  ½ large sweet red pepper, cubed
  ¼ large onion, thickly sliced
1–2 jalapeño peppers, chopped (wear plastic gloves
      when handling)
    1 bunch young kale leaves, coarsely chopped
  ⅓ cup defatted chicken stock
    2 medium tomatoes, coarsely chopped
    1 tablespoon balsamic vinegar
  ½ teaspoon grated orange peel
    2 tablespoons orange juice
  ½ teaspoon ground black pepper

Scrub the sweet potatoes and boil or microwave until just tender. Set aside until cool enough to handle. Remove the skins and thickly slice the flesh. Set aside.

While the sweet potatoes are cooking, place the oil in a 2½- or 3-quart ovenproof pot. Add the red peppers, onions and jalapeño peppers and stir to coat the vegetables with the oil. Roast at 450° for 5 to 7 minutes, or until the vegetables just begin to sizzle and brown. (Watch to make sure they don't burn.)

Stir in the kale to coat it evenly with oil and mix it with the vegetables. It will begin to wilt immediately. Top with the sweet-potato slices. Sprinkle with the stock.

Cover the casserole and braise on the stove top over medium-high heat until the kale is just cooked but still bright green, which should take about 5 minutes.

In a small bowl, mix the tomatoes, vinegar, orange peel, orange juice and black pepper. Evenly distribute over the vegetables in the casserole. Serve immediately.

Serves 4.

Per serving: 297 calories, 8.1 g. fat (25% of calories), 7.9 g. dietary fiber, 5.6 g. protein, 53.7 g. carbohydrates, 0 mg. cholesterol, 60 mg. sodium. Also a very good source of vitamins A, B_6, C and E.

Second Prize: Roberta A. Santangelo, St. Louis, Missouri

Roberta says she loves chocolate and she loves to cook! In addition to creating new recipes like this one, she makes over family favorites to cut the fat. This incredible recipe combines two all-American favorites—chocolate cake and apple pie—without all the fat and calories.

CHOCOLATE APPLE-PIE CAKE

CAKE

  1 **cup unbleached flour**
  2 **tablespoons cocoa powder**
  1 **teaspoon baking powder**
  1 **teaspoon baking soda**
  ¼ **cup chopped walnuts (optional)**
  ⅓ **cup skim milk**
  1 **tablespoon white vinegar**
  ⅔ **cup unsweetened applesauce**
  ½ **cup honey**
  3 **egg whites**
  3 **tablespoons + 1 teaspoon Crisco Puritan Oil**
  1 **teaspoon vanilla**

APPLE TOPPING

  2 **cups peeled and diced apples**
  ½ **cup orange juice**
  3 **tablespoons water**
  1 **tablespoon cornstarch**
  3 **large graham crackers, crushed into crumbs**
  1 **teaspoon ground cinnamon**

To make the cake: In a small bowl, thoroughly mix the flour, cocoa powder, baking powder and baking soda. Stir in the walnuts, if using.

In a cup, combine the milk and vinegar.

In a large bowl, beat together the applesauce, honey, egg

whites, oil, vanilla and the milk mixture with an electric mixer on low speed. Stir in the flour mixture and mix well. Coat an 8 × 8-inch baking pan with no-stick spray. Add the batter and bake at 350° for 35 to 40 minutes, or until a toothpick inserted in the center comes out clean. Let cool for 5 minutes before adding the topping.

To make the apple topping: While the cake is baking, combine the apples and orange juice in a 2-quart saucepan. Cover and cook over medium heat for 3 to 4 minutes, or until the apples are tender.

In a cup, mix the water and cornstarch. Pour into the pan with the apples and cook for about 1 minute, or until slightly thickened. Set aside to cool until needed.

When the cake is ready, spread the topping over it. Sprinkle with the graham crackers and cinnamon. Broil about 2 inches from the heat for 1 to 2 minutes; watch carefully so the topping doesn't burn.

Serves 12.

Per serving: 162 calories, 4.5 g. fat (24% of calories), 0.7 g. dietary fiber, 2.7 g. protein, 28.5 g. carbohydrates, 0 mg. cholesterol, 131 mg. sodium.

Third Prize: Pamela J. Stearns, Lakewood, California
Southern California and *Prevention* were Pamela's inspirations for this innovative recipe. As one of our testers said, it's "every person's breakfast with a twist" and a spicy kick.
Serve with salsa, melon balls and toast. Drizzle the toast with honey.

SOUTHWESTERN SUNDAY BRUNCH

SALSA

    5 large tomatoes, chopped
    1 onion, diced
    2 small Anaheim or other mild peppers, minced
    1 serrano or other hot pepper, minced (wear plastic gloves when handling)
    4 cloves garlic, minced
    2 tablespoons chopped fresh cilantro
    1 teaspoon red wine vinegar
       Pinch of ground black pepper

TORTILLA EGGS

    4 small flour tortillas
  2½ tablespoons Crisco Puritan Oil
    2 cups fat-free egg substitute
    2 strips turkey bacon, cooked and crumbled
   ¼ cup shredded reduced-fat Cheddar cheese (optional)

To make the salsa: In a medium bowl, combine the tomatoes, onions, mild peppers, hot peppers, garlic, cilantro, vinegar and black pepper. Chill.

To make the tortilla eggs: Cut the tortillas into thin strips ⅛ to ¼ inch wide and 2 inches long.

Place the oil in a large no-stick skillet and set over medium to medium-high heat until hot. Add the tortillas and cook, stirring, until golden brown; don't let the pieces burn. Drain on paper towels.

Lightly wipe out the skillet with paper towels, leaving a thin film of oil. Place over medium heat and add the egg substitute. Scramble according to the package directions. When the mixture is almost set, stir in the bacon and tortilla strips. Divide among individual plates. Sprinkle with the Cheddar, if using.

Serves 4.

Per serving: 522 calories, 14.4 g. fat (25% of calories), 7.9 g. dietary fiber, 21.6 g. protein, 81.7 g. carbohydrates, 5 mg. cholesterol, 524 mg. sodium. Also a very good source of thiamine, vitamin C, potassium and selenium.

Make It with Yogurt

SPONSORED BY DANNON

First Prize (in category) and Second Runner-Up Grand Prize: Mary Louise Lever, Rome, Georgia

Cool, creamy, calcium-rich and fruity is the perfect way to describe this warm-weather treat. With its mixture of yogurt, fruits and spices, this recipe makes a delicious cold bisque that one of our testers liked so much that she said "I could have eaten a gallon."

Mary Louise, an avid watercolorist, has found that she can "paint" with food. "I think fine food is an art," she says. "The thing that I love about cooking is not only does it have to taste good, I want the presentation to be pretty as well."

As the chairperson of the Floyd College Foundation in Rome, Georgia, Mary Louise has spiced up board meetings since she recruited members to sample her creations. "I'm their resident chef and chairperson," she said.

Mary Louise is no stranger to nutrition and healthy eating. When she was a little girl, her aunt owned one of the first health-food stores in Atlanta, where she also saw her first copy of *Prevention*. Mary Louise also makes it a point to exercise. She does aerobics and lifts weights three times a week at her local YMCA and also enjoys walking.

CHILLED CARIBBEAN FRUIT BISQUE WITH CINNAMON CRISPS

BISQUE

4	cups Dannon Plain Low-Fat Yogurt
4	large bananas, sliced (about 3 cups)
1½	teaspoons grated fresh ginger
¼	teaspoon ground cinnamon
1	can (8 ounces) crushed pineapple (with juice)
¾	teaspoon finely snipped fresh basil leaves

CINNAMON CRISPS

      4 **slices raisin bread**
    2½ **teaspoons reduced-fat corn-oil margarine, melted**
      ½ **teaspoon ground cinnamon**
      4 **large strawberries (garnish)**
         Basil sprigs (garnish)

To make the bisque: Place the yogurt, bananas, ginger and cinnamon in a blender. Process until smooth. Add the pineapple (with juice) and blend with several on/off turns until the pineapple is incorporated but not pureed. Stir in the basil.

Pour into a large bowl, cover and chill for at least 2 hours.

To make the cinnamon crisps: Trim the crusts from the bread. Cut the bread into ½-inch cubes. Place in a medium bowl.

In a small bowl, mix the margarine and cinnamon. Drizzle over the bread and toss to coat well.

Spread the bread in a single layer on a no-stick baking sheet and bake at 400° for 6 to 8 minutes, or until crisp and golden. Cool.

Serve the bisque topped with the crisps and garnished with the strawberries and basil sprigs.

Serves 4.

Per serving: 363 calories, 6.6 g. fat (16% of calories), 2.8 g. dietary fiber, 15.4 g. protein, 64 g. carbohydrates, 14 mg. cholesterol, 268 mg. sodium. Also a very good source of riboflavin, vitamins B_6 and B_{12}, calcium and potassium.

Second Prize: Lisa Keys, Middlebury, Connecticut

You can't go wrong with this flavorful dessert. With only 10 percent of calories from fat, this recipe is a great lifesaver when your sweet tooth is aching for a treat.

Healthy eating and exercise have helped Lisa keep up with her two active children. "It makes me look and feel great, and I can play tag for hours," she says.

GOLDEN APPLE-CRISP CUSTARD

4 cups sliced peeled apples
   Grated peel and juice of ½ lemon
3 tablespoons honey, divided
1 cup Dannon Vanilla Low-Fat Yogurt
¾ cup fat-free egg substitute
1 cup low-fat granola

Coat a 10-inch quiche dish or pie plate with no-stick spray.

In a large bowl, toss together the apples, lemon peel, lemon juice and 1 tablespoon of the honey. Spread in the prepared dish.

In the same bowl, whisk together the yogurt, egg substitute and the remaining 2 tablespoons honey. Pour over the apples.

Sprinkle with the granola, leaving a 1-inch rim around the edge. Bake at 350° for 50 to 60 minutes, or until puffed and golden. Serve warm.

Serves 8.

Per serving: 156 calories, 1.7 g. fat (10% of calories), 2.1 g. dietary fiber, 5 g. protein, 32.6 g. carbohydrates, 2 mg. cholesterol, 80 mg. sodium.

Third Prize: Larry Elder, Charlotte, North Carolina

Larry is interested in eating a low-fat, high-fiber diet, but it has to taste great, be exciting and be easy to prepare. This dish meets those requirements hands down, and the robust flavors really give your taste buds something to rave about.

CARIBBEAN JERK CHICKEN PAN PIZZA

1 tablespoon canola oil
1 cup cornmeal
¾ cup Dannon Plain Nonfat Yogurt
1 teaspoon ground cumin
2 cups diced cooked chicken breast
1 cup low-fat salsa
2 tablespoons Worcestershire sauce
1 tablespoon lime juice
½ teaspoon dried thyme
¼ teaspoon ground allspice
½ cup shredded reduced-fat Monterey Jack cheese
  with jalapeño peppers (see Note)
¼ cup chopped scallions
¼ cup diced sweet red peppers

Brush a large cast-iron skillet or other heavy ovenproof skillet with the oil. Bake at 400° for 5 minutes, or until hot.

In a small bowl, mix the cornmeal, yogurt and cumin. Carefully remove the pan from the oven and spoon the cornmeal mixture into it, spreading it evenly over the bottom.

Bake for 10 to 15 minutes, or until just firm and set but not browned. Remove from the oven.

In a medium bowl, mix the chicken, salsa, Worcestershire sauce, lime juice, thyme and allspice. Spread evenly over the cornmeal mixture. Sprinkle with the Monterey Jack, scallions and peppers. Bake for 10 to 12 minutes, or until bubbly.

Note: You may substitute plain Monterey Jack cheese and 2 tablespoons minced fresh or canned jalapeño peppers.

Serves 4.

Per serving: 319 calories, 8.5 g. fat (24% of calories), 5 g. dietary fiber, 26.7 g. protein, 34.2 g. carbohydrates, 47 mg. cholesterol, 865 mg. sodium. Also a very good source of niacin and vitamins A and C.

Make It with Rice

Sᴘᴏɴsᴏʀᴇᴅ ʙʏ Mᴀʜᴀᴛᴍᴀ, Sᴜᴄᴄᴇss, Cᴀʀᴏʟɪɴᴀ ᴀɴᴅ Rɪᴠᴇʀ Bʀᴏᴡɴ Rɪᴄᴇ

First Prize: Annemarie Westfall-Ferrero, Marina Del Rey, California

Annemarie grew up on this dish, which had been passed down from generation to generation in Germany until she brought it to the United States.

In fact, it was her desire to share the recipe with others that inspired her to enter our contest.

With apples, raisins and lemon, this dish offers a burst of flavor that can be served hot or cold. It's so versatile that you can eat it for breakfast, lunch or dinner as well as a snack or dessert.

Surprisingly, for all its great taste, this soufflé gets only 6 percent of its calories from fat.

Working as a medical social worker at Kaiser-Permanente and taking classes in applied psychology at the University of Santa Monica keep Annemarie pretty busy. On weekends, she looks forward to walks on the beach and experimenting with new recipes.

Aɴɴᴇᴍᴀʀɪᴇ's Gᴇʀᴍᴀɴ Aᴘᴘʟᴇ-Rɪᴄᴇ Sᴏᴜꜰꜰʟé

- ¾ cup Carolina Extra Long Grain Enriched Rice
- 1 egg, separated, or 2 egg whites
- 3 tablespoons honey
  Grated peel of ½ lemon
- 1 apple, peeled and diced
- ¼ cup raisins
- ¼ teaspoon vanilla, rum or brandy extract

Bring a large pot of water to a boil. Add the rice and cook over medium-low heat for 14 minutes, or until tender. Drain and rinse briefly with cold water. Set aside.

Place 1 egg white in a small bowl and beat with an electric mixer until stiff.

Place the egg yolk or remaining egg white in a large bowl. Add the honey and lemon peel. Beat with an electric mixer for about 3 minutes. Fold in the rice, apples, raisins and extract.

Fold in the beaten egg white.

Coat a 1½-quart casserole with no-stick spray. Add the rice mixture. Bake at 350° for 25 to 30 minutes, or until set. Serve hot or cold.

Serves 4.

Per serving: 243 calories, 1.7 g. fat (6% of calories), 1.6 g. dietary fiber, 4.4 g. protein, 53.4 g. carbohydrates, 53 mg. cholesterol, 20 mg. sodium.

Second Prize: Gloria Bradley, Naperville, Illinois

Since her husband had a heart attack last year, Gloria said they completely changed their way of eating. In an effort to cut fat, she has been using more turkey, vegetables and rice. It's working! This dish has a very low 19 percent of calories from fat, with 100 percent taste.

Tex-Mex Turkey, Rice and Lime Stew

¾ cup River Natural Long Grain Brown Rice
1 can (13¾ ounces) defatted reduced-sodium chicken stock
1 can (14½ ounces) no-salt-added tomatoes, chopped
½ cup minced onions
3–4 jalapeño peppers, minced (wear plastic gloves when handling)
¼ teaspoon ground cumin
¼ teaspoon chili powder
1½ cups cubed cooked turkey breast
1 package (10 ounces) frozen corn
2 tablespoons lime juice
1 cup shredded reduced-fat Monterey Jack cheese
¼ cup crushed tortilla chips

In a 2-quart saucepan over medium heat, bring 2 cups of water to a boil. Add the rice. Reduce the heat to medium-low, cover the pan and cook for 35 to 45 minutes, or until the rice is tender and all the liquid has been absorbed. Fluff with a fork and keep warm.

In a 3-quart saucepan, combine the stock, tomatoes, onions, peppers, cumin and chili powder. Bring to a boil. Reduce the heat and simmer for 10 minutes. Stir in the turkey, corn, lime juice and rice. Simmer for 5 minutes, or until heated through.

To serve, ladle into bowls. Sprinkle with the Monterey Jack and tortilla chips.

Serves 4.

Per serving: 422 calories, 9 g. fat (19% of calories), 5.3 g. dietary fiber, 31.6 g. protein, 56.8 g. carbohydrates, 36 mg. cholesterol, 519 mg. sodium. Also a very good source of niacin and vitamins A, B$_6$ and C.

Third Prize: Narayanachar Murali, M.D., Lexington, Kentucky

This hearty dish is packed with vitamins, minerals and fiber—and it's low in fat. As a doctor, Narayanachar knows the benefits of healthy eating, and with this recipe, he's setting an excellent example.

SPINACH AND LENTIL PULLAO WITH RAITA

PULLAO

> 5 teaspoons canola oil
> ½ teaspoon black mustard seeds
> 3 cups finely chopped spinach
> 1 cup lentils, soaked overnight, drained and patted dry
> 2–3 hot green chili peppers, seeded and julienned (wear plastic gloves when handling)
> ¼ cup raisins
> ½ teaspoon finely chopped fresh ginger
> 1½ cups Mahatma or Carolina Extra Long Grain Enriched Rice
> 1 teaspoon curry powder
> Pinch of turmeric
> 2½ cups boiling water

RAITA

> 1 bag (16 ounces) frozen mixed vegetables
> 1 teaspoon canola oil
> ⅛ teaspoon cumin seeds
> 1 teaspoon curry powder
> 1 cup plain nonfat yogurt
> 2 tablespoons buttermilk
> ½ cup diced tomatoes
> ¼ cup chopped fresh cilantro

To make the pullao: In a Dutch oven over medium heat, warm the oil. Add the mustard seeds and cook for 30 seconds. Add the spinach, lentils, peppers, raisins and ginger. Sauté for 5 minutes.

Add the rice and sauté, stirring constantly, for 5 to 6 minutes. Stir in the curry powder and turmeric. Add the water. Cover and cook over medium-low heat for 20 minutes, or until the rice and lentils are tender.

To make the raita: While the rice is cooking, place the frozen vegetables in a strainer and rinse with hot water to thaw them. Drain well and pat dry.

Place the oil in a 2-quart saucepan and warm over medium heat. Add the cumin seeds and cook for about 30 seconds, or until the seeds begin crackling. Add the vegetables and cook over medium-low heat for 5 minutes. Stir in the curry powder. Cool for about 30 minutes.

Transfer to a medium bowl. Stir in the yogurt and buttermilk. Sprinkle with the tomatoes and cilantro. Serve with the rice.

Serves 4.

Per serving: 624 calories, 8.6 g. fat (12% of calories), 11 g. dietary fiber, 27.1 g. protein, 113 g. carbohydrates, 1 mg. cholesterol, 136 mg. sodium. Also a very good source of thiamine, folate, vitamins A and C, iron, magnesium and potassium.

Mediterranean Magic

Fresh vegetables, fragrant herbs and a good dose of olive oil make this French cuisine savory and healthy.

Drive south, down the long, dull auto route from Paris, and just above the old walled city of Avignon, you have your first awakening sense of France's Mediterranean region—the sense of smell. The permeating sweetness of lavender, the pungent odors of herbs—thyme, oregano, rosemary—waft sweet in the air. Then the eyes widen as fields of hazy purple-gray lavender, endless bushes of tufted yellow broom and swathes of sunflowers pass by, and the ears listen attentively to that loud buzzing of cicadas.

If ever God created a more beautiful land than this to soothe the soul and nourish all the senses, I have never found it. And if a more glorious regional cuisine exists, I have never tasted it. Sprung from the herbs rooted in the rocky soil, the olive trees twisted and gnarled on the terraced hillsides, netted from the Mediterranean that laps along the shore of France from Nice to Marseilles, this food is bright and flavorful, glossy with olive oil, full of sun and sea and heady with garlic, always garlic.

Spend time in this southernmost reach of France, which is called Provence, and it's easy to see how the area gave rise to a unique cuisine. I always think of pure, healthy fruits and vegetables picked in their prime, sold in the open-air markets and served at home with pristine perfection: the tiny parboiled green beans dressed only with olive oil and a drop of vinegar; the small orange melons, rich with perfume, on which you can make a lunch; the dark red cherries that you eat with green, cracked-open almonds always for dessert. Breakfast typically is fresh-pressed juice, brewed coffee and slabs of grilled whole-grain peasant bread with apricot home preserves.

Travel to Provence, and you cannot soon help feeling healthier, more vital than when you came. You adapt to siestas—and the natural need for them after a large lunch on a hot day. Shop hours, after all, cease for a three-hour period each afternoon, then extend into early evening when the day cools. You buy a pair of espadrilles, rope-soled canvas shoes, and clamber up and down the terraces and mazy cobbled streets, and soon, like the rest of the people who live here, you have wiry, well-developed calves and thighs. You buy a mesh bag and walk to market most every day to purchase exquisitely fresh vegetables and fruits and your just-baked daily bread.

Shopping for Lunch

Rise early, carry four empty mesh bags and walk down to the port area of Toulon, the ancient naval city in southeastern Provence. Vendors have been up since 6:00 A.M., setting up their market wares along 20 blocks. Giant plane trees shade the street, and the cries of the sellers challenge the customers to feel, smell, sample-taste and buy.

First to the fishmongers for a good grilling fish. Masses of little, brightly colored fish are on the stands today. A huge tuna rests between sawhorses, and two men, using a double-handled saw, slice back and forth. We select a delicate-flavored fish to grill in the Provençal manner.

We pass the olive vendor, where we buy pure pressed oil and then choose from the multitude of briny barrels some herb-marinated small olives. The variety of mixed lettuces and sharp rustic greens (for example, mesclun) is irresistible, as are radishes, luscious figs and the soft white, made-that-morning cheese, for our simple alfresco luncheon at home.

Easing the Pace

The pace of life in Provence is slower, more measured than in America. Lunchtimes stretch for two hours. Time at the table is spent conversing.

In hot weather, there is always a respite nap after lunch. People tend to eat lightly at supper on an everyday basis, though there are some large, heavy restaurant meals on special occasions.

People who live in Provence take time off in the month of August, as do the rest of their fellow countrymen. It is necessary, therapeutic to the soul. Some go to spas, others camp in the fresh air of the mountains or at the seashore. Or they simply take days off for excursions. They might drive to a honey-vendor's stand or visit a local wine maker.

Family Gatherings at the Beach

There is time in August for familial gatherings. Frequently, someone brings all the elements of a bouillabaisse (BOOL-yuh-BAYZ), a saffron-flavored fish stew, and its from-scratch cooking provides an afternoon's entertainment. The children dig a hole in the sand and gather driftwood for a fire. The men tend the fire. Elderly ladies peel potatoes; the younger women make hot, peppery rouille (rou-EE) sauce to add to the stew and cut slices of bread to dry so that they can absorb more delicious fish stock.

Onions, tomatoes, saffron and herbs cook down in seawater. Potato slices and thick fillets of fish go on top, then later delicate little fish are added at the last moment. The fire is fierce. Bouillabaisse is always waited for. Patience is required. At the precise moment of perfection, all must be seated at the table. Later, the plates are dipped in the sea and stacked in picnic baskets to be carried back in the boat. If there is any leftover bouillabaisse, it is carried home, any fish bones are picked out, and it is placed in a small bowl. The gelatin from the fish bones will solidify the remains, and the next day, jellied cold bouillabaisse is sliced and eaten for lunch.

Waste Not

This is the kind of frugality common to the area. Little gets wasted. People recycle simple ingredients from one dish into the next if there are leftovers, and of course, daily marketing means frugal purchasing. It is common to put leftover green beans (perhaps last night's supper) into a composed salad of greens, tomatoes and herbs.

Leftovers are collected, then added to soupe au pistou, a kind of vegetable soup thickened with small noodles into which each person then stirs spoonfuls of basil and garlic pistou (pesto) sauce.

One trait of Provençal meals that I especially appreciate is how often they encourage personal involvement on the diner's part. Children and older people alike "play with their food." Fava beans are split open with the fingers, then the beans are taken out and dipped into seasonings.

A Provençal Lunch

First course: radishes, olives, fresh bread and olive oil.
The French can make a whole course of radishes and olives.
Clean and trim radishes, but leave an inch of green leaves on
top for a handle. Place the radishes in a small rustic bowl.
Place small olives in another bowl and add a bay leaf and
thyme sprigs for garnish. Each person needs a small bowl of
olive oil. Everyone dips chunks of fresh bread into the oil.
Alternate bites of radishes, olives and bread. Eat slowly.
Converse pleasantly.

**Second course: grilled whole fish (such as red snapper)
with fennel.** Walk up the nearest hillside and cut down
branches of wild fennel weed. Failing that, buy bulb fennel.
Slice the tender white hearts into a salad, but use the stalks
and feathery tops for your fish. Mince a tablespoon of feathery
top greens. Pour a liberal amount of olive oil over the fish, rub
in the chopped fennel and leave the fish to marinate, refriger-
ated, for one hour.

Heat the grill. Grill the fish, and while it is on the fire, dip

Guests often slip a knife under their plates to tilt them,
then make their own vinaigrette sauce from the olive-oil
bottle and the vinegar cruet on the table. They eat commu-
nally from the big platter of slender green beans that were
steamed al dente, each person dipping beans into his own
sauce. Artichokes are a common first course that also involve hand labor, and thus a longer, more relaxed and intimate time at table.

Often, the cook or host prepares one of Provence's famous dipping sauces right at the table. Rouille and pistou
are two regional sauces that might appear on the table,

a stalk of fennel into the marinade oil and brush the fish frequently.

Eat with bread. Pick the fish slowly from the bone. Converse intelligently.

Salad: mixed greens. Choose from an assortment of tender, young leaves like arugula (also known as rocket or roquette) and mâche. Dress lightly with a good olive oil and a splash of wine vinegar.

Dessert: white cheese with black cherries or figs. Cheese and fruit are the typical dessert in Provence. Brousse cheese, made from fresh sheep's milk in the predawn morning, is sold two days each week at the Toulon market. It is considered a great delicacy, similar to goat's cheese. As for figs, cut off the stems, then make two slices at right angles halfway down each fruit. Hold the fruit from the bottom, squeeze it open and gently suck the pink-seeded pulp off the skin, which any true connoisseur will then discard. Converse tenderly when you eat figs.

along with a platter of assorted vegetables and fresh bread, to be used for dipping.

Celebrating Garlic

Once a year in the summertime, whole small towns in Provence take the afternoon off to celebrate their own communities and to celebrate garlic. That garlic is revered in Provence, that it marries so beautifully with herbs and olive oil and that it is an intrinsic part of most famous dishes comes as no surprise when you visit the area. Garlic vendors, their bicycles laden with strings of garlic, pass through villages as soon as the new crop has been cut each September. Ropes of garlic hang in every Provençal kitchen. Any dish worthy of the name à la Provençal had better contain tomatoes, herbs and a good slug of garlic.

VEGETABLE SOUP WITH PISTOU

This Provençal minestrone, properly known as soupe au pistou, is an ideal way to use up leftovers—traditionally potatoes, tomatoes, zucchini, carrots, winter squash and at least two types of beans. A bowl of pistou is kept on the table so spoonfuls can be swirled into the soup. Grated Parmesan is also usually on the table so diners can sprinkle some onto the soup. Complete the meal with bread and fruit.

>   2   **cups cooked white beans**
>   2   **cups peeled, cubed potatoes**
>   2   **cups tomato wedges**
>   1   **cup sliced carrots**
>   1   **cup sliced leeks**
>   1   **cup sliced onions**
>   1   **cup sliced zucchini**
>   1   **cup cubed pumpkin or butternut squash**
>   1   **cup halved green beans**
>   2   **tablespoons chopped fresh parsley**
>   1   **teaspoon dried thyme**
>   1   **clove garlic, minced**
>   **Ground black pepper, to taste**
>   **Pinch of ground red pepper**
>   2   **ounces vermicelli or other thin pasta, broken**
>   **into 2-inch pieces**
>   6   **tablespoons pistou (see recipe on the opposite page)**

In a Dutch oven or other large pot, combine the white beans, potatoes, tomatoes, carrots, leeks, onions, zucchini, pumpkin or squash, green beans, parsley, thyme, garlic and black and red pepper. Add enough cold water to cover the vegetables by about 2 inches.

Bring to a boil. Reduce the heat and simmer for 20 minutes, or until the vegetables are almost tender. Add the pasta. Simmer for another 10 minutes, or until the pasta is cooked and the vegetables are tender.

Ladle into bowls and serve with the pistou.

Serves 6.

Per serving: 253 calories, 4.9 grams fat (2.3 g. monounsaturated fat), 5.9 g. dietary fiber, 10.8 g. protein, 44.2 g. carbohydrates, 2 mg. cholesterol, 80 mg. sodium. Also a good source of vitamins A, B₆ and C and potassium.

PISTOU

This is the French version of pesto sauce. It's an excellent way to store a bumper basil crop. Store it in the refrigerator, where it will keep for a month. Like rouille, pistou will separate during storage. Simply stir it well before using.

> **2 cups loosely packed basil leaves**
> **3–4 cloves garlic, minced**
> **2 tablespoons pine nuts**
> **¼ cup olive oil**
> **½ cup grated Parmesan or finely shredded Gruyère cheese**

In a food processor, combine the basil, garlic and pine nuts. Process with on/off turns until finely chopped. (Add a little oil as necessary to make blending easier.)

Transfer to a bowl. Thoroughly stir in the oil and Parmesan or Gruyère to form a creamy sauce with the consistency of thick gravy.

Makes about 1¼ cups.

Per tablespoon: 43 calories, 4 g. fat (2.2 g. monounsaturated fat), 0.1 g. dietary fiber, 1.4 g. protein, 0.8 g. carbohydrates, 2 mg. cholesterol, 47 mg. sodium.

ROUILLE

This fiery dipping sauce is great with vegetables. Or stir spoonfuls of it into soups and fish stews.

> 1 **hot red pepper, seeds removed (wear plastic gloves when handling)**
> 3 **cloves garlic, chopped**
> 2 **slices firm bread, crusts removed**
> ⅓ **cup olive oil**
> **Ground black pepper, to taste**

Chop the red pepper. Using a mini food processor or a mortar and pestle, thoroughly crush the peppers and garlic into a paste.

Hold the bread under cold running water. When it is soaked, squeeze out the moisture. Add the bread to the food processor or mortar and blend well.

Slowly blend in the oil to form a sauce of medium consistency. Add the black pepper.

Makes about ½ cup.

Per tablespoon: 97 calories, 9.2 g. fat (6.7 g. monounsaturated fat), 0.1 g. dietary fiber, 0.6 g. protein, 3.3 g. carbohydrates, 0 g. cholesterol, 30 mg. sodium.

FRENCH ONION TART

The French call it pissaladière (pee-sah-lah-DYAIR). It's the thin, crisp, onion-laden pizza of Provence. And it's sold whole or by the slice in bakeries and marketplaces. You can make it on a base of pizza dough, standard bread dough or even pie dough flavored with olive oil. If using yeast dough, allow it to rise once. While the standard shape is round, ovals and free-form tarts are handsome and rustic. The olives traditionally used are the tiny black Niçoise variety. They have a relatively

large stone for their size, so warn diners not to bite down hard
on them.

> 3 **large onions, chopped**
> ¼ **cup olive oil, divided**
> ¼ **teaspoon dried thyme**
>   **Bread dough or pastry (enough to make a**
>   **12-inch crust)**
> 2 **tins anchovies**
> ⅓ **cup Niçoise olives**

Combine the onions and 3 tablespoons of the oil in a
large, heavy frying pan. Cook over low heat, stirring frequently, for 20 minutes, or until the onions turn a rich gold
color and are very soft. About halfway through the cooking
period, stir in the thyme.

Pat or roll the dough or pastry into a round or oval about
¼ inch thick. Spray a pizza pan or large baking sheet with
no-stick spray and place the dough on it. Turn up the edges
to form a small rim.

Spread the onions evenly over the surface. Drain the
anchovies and pat the fillets dry on paper towels. Arrange
the anchovies in a grid pattern over the onions. Place an
olive in the center of each square.

Sprinkle lightly with the remaining 1 tablespoon oil. Bake
at 400° for 15 to 20 minutes, or until the crust is golden on
the bottom.

Serves 6.

*Per serving: 385 calories, 11.2 g. fat (7.2 g. monounsaturated fat), 6.6 g.
dietary fiber, 12.2 g. protein, 60.5 g. carbohydrates, 7 mg. cholesterol, 356
mg. sodium. Also a good source of thiamine and folate.*

GARLIC BROTH

In France, garlic is considered more than a food; it's a restorative, as good for the body as it is for the soul. Garlic equals good taste and good medicine, as in this broth.

6 **cloves garlic**
2 **cups water**
1 **bay leaf**
1 **tablespoon olive oil**
2 **fresh sage leaves**

Peel and slice the garlic. Place in a 1-quart saucepan along with the water, bay leaf, oil and sage leaves. Bring to a boil and simmer for 15 minutes. Strain and serve in mugs. Sip slowly and inhale the fragrance.

Serves 2.

Per serving: 60 calories, 6.9 g. fat (5 g. monounsaturated fat).

SOURCE: Judith Olney, a restaurant critic for the *Washington Times* and author of six cookbooks, including *Comforting Food* and *The Farm Market Cookbook*, has spent many summers in Toulon, in the south of France, savoring the Mediterranean way of life.

Credits

"Find the Body Weight That's Best for You" on page 14 was adapted from "Balancing Act" by Liz Applegate, Ph.D. Copyright © 1993 by Liz Applegate, Ph.D. Reprinted by permission.

"Ten Surefire Tricks to Help You Stay on Your Diet" on page 19 was adapted from an article by Gwenda Blair originally published in *SELF* magazine. Copyright © 1994 by Gwenda Blair. Reprinted by permission.

"The Truth about Dieting" on page 25 was adapted from "Lifting Weight Myths" by David Schardt. Copyright © 1993, Center for Science in the Public Interest. Adapted from *Nutrition Action Healthletter* (1875 Connecticut Avenue NW, Suite 300, Washington, DC 20009-5728. $24.00 for 10 issues).

"Another Side of Beef" by Jim Thornton on page 73 was adapted from an article originally published in *Men's Health*. Copyright © 1994 by Jim Thornton. Reprinted by permission.

"The Deskside Stretch" on page 177 was excerpted from *Computer and Desk Stretches* by Robert A. Anderson and Jean E. Anderson. Copyright © 1986. For a free catalog of other publications, contact Stretching Inc., P.O. Box 767, Palmer Lake, CO 80133; 1-800-333-1307.

"Walk This Way" on page 184 was adapted from "The Way You Walk" by Judith Stone that was originally published in *HEALTH*. Copyright © 1994. Reprinted by permission from *HEALTH*.

"Five Hot New Ways to Stay Fit" by David Higdon on page 215 was adapted from an article originally published in *SELF* magazine. Copyright © 1994 by David Higdon. Reprinted by permission.

Index